OZEMPIC

RISKS, BENEFITS, AND NATURAL ALTERNATIVES TO GLP-1 WEIGHT-LOSS DRUGS

Michael Greger, M.D., FACLM

New York Times Bestselling Author of *How Not to Die*, *How Not to Diet*, and *How Not to Age*

Founder of NutritionFacts.org

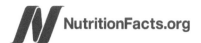

Also by Michael Greger, M.D., FACLM

How Not to Die

The How Not to Die Cookbook

How Not to Diet

The How Not to Diet Cookbook

How to Survive a Pandemic

How Not to Age

OZEMPIC: RISKS, BENEFITS, AND NATURAL ALTERNATIVES TO GLP-1 WEIGHT-LOSS DRUGS. Copyright © 2024 by NutritionFacts.org Inc. All rights reserved. Printed in the United States of America. For information, address NutritionFacts.org, P.O. Box 11400, Takoma Park, MD 20913.

NutritionFacts.org

The Library of Congress Catologing-in-Publication Data is available upon request.

LCCN 2024920656
ISBN 979-8-9916605-0-1 (paperback)
ISBN 979-8-9916605-1-8 (e-book)

First paperback edition, October 2024

Book design, cover art, graphs, and charts by Caroline Garriott, NutritionFacts.org

CONTENTS

INTRODUCTION

Ozempic and others in a new class of weight-loss drugs have received enormous, almost unprecedented attention in the mainstream media.[1] They have been called "the medical sensation of the decade,"[2] and the business press has been practically giddy, boldly declaring "the end of obesity."[3]

The enthusiasm has been shared in the medical literature, where headlines suggest they are "game changers,"[4] "a revolution in the treatment of obesity,"[5] "therapeutic wizard[s],"[6] and "miracle drugs"[7] that "are hugely effective"[8] in treating obesity.

What are these purported panaceas? A naturally occurring hormone in our body called *glucagon-like peptide-1* (GLP-1) plays a role in regulating our blood sugar, appetite, and digestion, and these new anti-obesity drugs are GLP-1 *agonists*, meaning they mimic the action of the hormone by binding to GLP-1 receptors.[9] Are they worthy of all this hype?

Magic Bullets or Blanks (or Worse)

History is littered with failed weight-loss wonder drugs. Every other year or so, an anti-obesity medication that had been approved as safe and effective has had to be withdrawn from the marketplace after the emergence of serious side effects.[10] From "rainbow diet pills" packed with amphetamines marketed to 1950s housewives to the rise and fall of fen-phen,[11] the vast majority of weight-loss drugs approved in the United States have been pulled from the market for unforeseen side effects[12] that turned them into a public health threat.[13]

The appetite suppressant aminorex, for example, was widely prescribed before being pulled for causing lung damage.[14] Eighteen million Americans were on fen-phen before it was pulled[15] for causing severe damage to heart valves.[16] Meridia was pulled for heart attacks and strokes,[17] and Acomplia for psychiatric side effects, including suicide.[18]

Lorcaserin, sold as Belviq, was withdrawn in 2020 after it was recognized that it may have been causing cancer for the eight years it had been on the market.[19] The U.S. Food and Drug Administration (FDA) had initially rejected it after it appeared to cause several kinds of tumors in rats, but when a one-year human trial showed no apparent cancer issues, it gained FDA approval and became one of the most frequently prescribed weight-loss medications. After people took it for a few years, though, notably high rates of colorectal cancer, pancreatic cancer, and lung cancer started to emerge, so it was eventually pulled.[20] This reversal was "met with surprise and confusion among obesity medicine specialists," the journal *Obesity* editorialized. "It was particularly jarring because this drug was generally regarded as having a favorable tolerability and safety profile with a positive effect on hyperglycemia."[21] It was considered safe, until it wasn't.

Historically, losing weight with pills has been like losing weight with puffs. Like cigarettes, anti-obesity drugs can make you thinner, but at what cost?[22] The goal of weight loss is not to fit into a skinnier casket.

One Pill Makes You Small

There are several drug options currently on the market. Qsymia is a combination of phentermine, the *phen* in fen-phen, and topiramate, a drug that can cause seizures if you abruptly stop taking it.[23] It was explicitly rejected multiple times for safety reasons in Europe but remains for sale in the United States. Naltrexone/bupropion, sold as Contrave, is another possibility if you choose to ignore its black box warning about a potential increase in suicidal thoughts.[24] And there's orlistat, sold as Alli and Xenical, which blocks fat absorption, causes side effects such as "flatus with discharge,"[25] and evidently "forces the patient to use diapers and to know the location of all the bathrooms in the neighborhood in an attempt to limit the consequences of urgent leakage of oily fecal matter"[26]—all for just a 3 percent loss in body weight.[27]

Overall, older weight-loss medications achieved about 5 percent weight loss.[28] As a class, GLP-1 agonists only average 6 percent, but that includes some of the older drugs, like liraglutide and exenatide, which are less effective. Semaglutide, which is sold as Ozempic for diabetes or Wegovy for weight loss, causes about twice that.[29] Then there's tirzepatide, sold as Mounjaro or Zepbound, which edges closer to what you might see with certain bariatric surgery procedures.[30] The reason these newer GLP-1 agonists are considered to be such game changers is that, while the older anti-obesity medications achieve weight losses in the 5 to 10 percent range, this new generation of GLP-1 mimics may reach 15 to 20 percent.[31]

So, while there has long been a healthy skepticism about each new "latest and greatest" anti-obesity drug that failed to deliver on its promises, these new drugs are positioned to topple the historical narrative that so reliably presumed the next flop, given their tripling of weight-loss efficacy over previous attempts.[32] But how well do these new GLP-1 agonist drugs really work? How do they work? For how long? What are the short-term side effects? The long-term side effects? Are there safer, cheaper, natural alternatives to boost GLP-1 with diet and lifestyle?

In this primer, I'll cut through the promotional puffery to lay out the pros and cons so individuals can make up their own mind in the face of the very real and devastating consequences of obesity.

WHAT IS GLP-1?

The gastrointestinal tract is known as the largest hormone-secreting gland in our body, and it releases more than 20 different peptide hormones. About 1 in every 100 cells lining our digestive tract acts as a nutrient sensor and can secrete hormones accordingly, including glucagon-like peptide-1.[33] The primary stimuli for secreting GLP-1 are meals rich in fats and carbohydrates,[34] and GLP-1's main action is to signal satiety to the brain.[35] This results in a reduction in our appetite so we don't eat too many donuts.

GLP-1 also slows down our digestion. Delaying the rate at which food leaves our stomach not only helps us feel fuller for longer, but it also helps with our blood sugar control.[36] In fact, GLP-1-mimicking drugs were first developed to treat diabetes.[37]

The Breakthrough in Lizard Spit

Why do we need a drug that *mimics* GLP-1? Can't we just take the hormone directly? No, because our body breaks down[38] GLP-1 so quickly that it hardly makes it even one time around our circulatory system.[39]

Then, a compound was discovered—in the venomous saliva of a lizard called the Gila monster[40]—that mimics GLP-1 but is resistant to breakdown.

Using that compound as a template, the first GLP-1 agonist was created and approved for the treatment of diabetes about 20 years ago. Instead of most of it being cleared from the body within two and a half minutes, like native, natural GLP-1, much of the drug remains in the body for two and a half hours. That still means twice-daily injections, though, so then came liraglutide, which lasts all day. Eventually, semaglutide was developed and branded as Ozempic, which could be injected just once a *week*.[41]

Ozempic was approved in 2017 to treat diabetes.[42] Within a few years, a daily oral version had been developed, again for diabetes, but researchers running those clinical trials noticed a surprising side effect: People's appetites diminished.[43] Indeed, when GLP-1 or an agonist is dripped into people's veins, appetite is reduced, leading to markedly reduced food consumption[44]—a decrease in caloric intake by as much as 25 to 50 percent.[45]

Benfluorex Cover-Up

Like Ozempic, benfluorex, sold as Mediator, was another drug created for diabetes that had been repurposed as an appetite suppressant. Despite causing hundreds of deaths, benfluorex didn't get pulled from the market for 33 years.[46] Its manufacturer knew about the drug's risks but covered them up. Judges concluded that the drug company's "priority was systematically given to preserving [its own] economic interests over the safety of the drug's consumers."[47] How many decades will pass before we understand the long-term effects of Ozempic?

Ozempic on the Brain

The GLP-1 hormone acts as an appetite suppressant by targeting parts of the brain responsible for hunger and cravings.[48] GLP-1-secreting cells don't only line our intestines; they're also in our brains.[49] So, in a way, GLP-1 agonist drugs work like birth control pills. The Pill mimics placental hormones, thereby tricking our body into thinking we're pregnant all the time.[50] Ozempic-type drugs mimic GLP-1, thereby tricking our body into thinking we're eating all the time. That's how it dials down our hunger drive.

Four years after semaglutide had been approved as Ozempic to treat diabetes, it was rebranded at a higher dose as Wegovy to treat obesity.[51] Overnight, the weight-loss industry changed, shifting from meal replacements and portion control plans to the new world of private equity–funded telemedicine entities offering injectable weight-loss drugs. Even Weight Watchers has openly embraced these types of drugs as the future of weight loss.[52] They were even approved for kids as young as age 12—tweens, not yet teens.[53]

HOW WELL DO GLP-1 DRUGS WORK?

Traditional weight-loss medications, like fen-phen's phentermine, achieved a reduction in body weight of about 5 percent over placebo,[54] whereas these new GLP-1 agonists, including semaglutide and tirzepatide, produce about triple the effect, around a 15 percent reduction.[55] What does that mean in terms of numbers on the bathroom scale?

In an analysis of more than a hundred clinical studies of earlier anti-obesity medications in trials lasting up to 76 weeks, drug-induced weight loss never exceeded more than nine pounds.[56] In contrast, putting together all the GLP-1 drug trials, which ran around 52 weeks on average, they led to about 19 pounds of weight loss.[57] However, that folded in results from some of the older GLP-1 drugs that don't work as well. Looking only at semaglutide, the high-dose Ozempic sold as Wegovy for weight loss, body-weight reduction was more like 27 pounds, which translates into about three and a half inches off the waist.[58]

Which GLP-1 drug works the best? An oral version of Ozempic has been developed,[59] but it hasn't yet been approved for weight loss. However, preliminary evidence suggests it causes similar weight loss to the injectable version.[60] Tirzepatide, sold as Mounjaro or Zepbound, is the latest with FDA approval as a weight-loss drug and appears to beat out semaglutide, resulting in about 45 pounds of weight loss and five and a half inches off the waist.[61]

Syringe vs. Scalpel

How do these results compare to bariatric surgery? They aren't that far off from what can be achieved with long-term surgical weight loss, but these are averages.[62] Bariatric surgery doesn't always work; the failure rate for the gold-standard procedure is approximately 20 percent.[63] But not everyone responds to GLP-1 drugs either.[64]

In the major semaglutide drug trials, about a third of study participants were "super responders," but as many as one in six didn't lose a significant amount of weight at all—even after taking the drug for more than a year.[65] Some patients can even *gain* dozens of pounds despite years on the drug.[66] So, despite impressive results at a population level, up to 20 percent of individuals fail to achieve significant weight loss with either surgical or drug-based approaches.[67]

The Weight-Loss Plateau

The vast majority do lose weight on the new GLP-1 drugs, but that weight loss stalls after about a year. In the longest trial to date, more than 17,000 individuals were randomized to injections of either high-dose semaglutide or placebo for four years.[68] Overall, those on the drug lost 9 percent more body weight than those in the placebo group, but all the weight was lost in the first 65 weeks. Even though they continued to get injected every week for three more years, they didn't lose any more weight over the subsequent 143 weeks.

This weight-loss plateau happened in study after study, not only for semaglutide, but also the newer GLP-1 drug, tirzepatide. So, even under the best of circumstances, with the most potent GLP-1 drugs taken at the highest allowable dose for at least a year to obtain the full weight-loss benefit before plateau, researchers have found only about a 34-pound drop before the weight loss stops.

In figure 1[69,70,71] are the weight-loss graphs of the three major placebo-controlled trials featured in the drug insert included in every package of high-dose semaglutide (Wegovy):

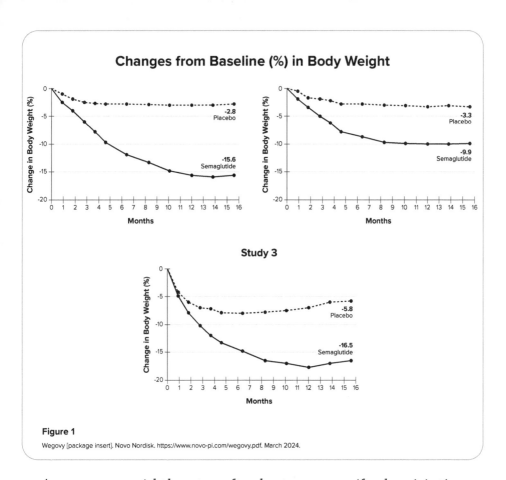

Figure 1

Wegovy [package insert]. Novo Nordisk. https://www.novo-pi.com/wegovy.pdf. March 2024.

As you can see, weight loss stops after about a year, even if we keep injecting ourselves with the drug. Is it because the study participants plateaued at a normal weight? Sadly, no, as you can see in figure 2.[72,73,74] They started out obese, and they ended up obese.

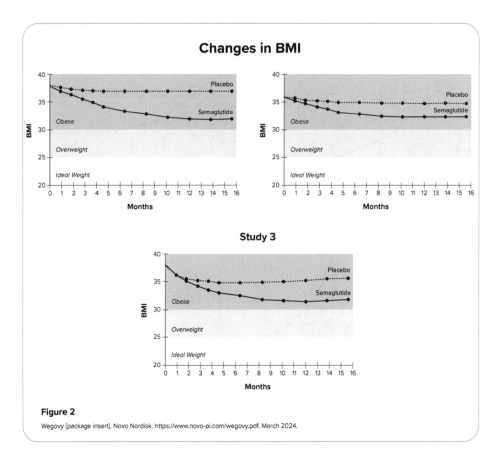

Figure 2

Wegovy [package insert]. Novo Nordisk. https://www.novo-pi.com/wegovy.pdf. March 2024.

These are the same graphs as figure 1, but they show weight status. At the start of the study, the participants were obese with an average body mass index (BMI) of about 37. After more than a year on the drug—after it effectively stops working—they were still obese with an average BMI of about 32. They were certainly less obese, but still obese.

Given the wide hype these drugs are getting, their limitations may not be understood.[75] The drugs don't work for everyone, and, even when they do work, weight loss stalls after a year, potentially still leaving individuals obese and feeling compelled to stay on the drugs for the rest of their lives for fear of regaining the original weight they lost.[76]

Why the Weight Loss Stops

Weight loss tends to plateau regardless of the method used to shed pounds. Why? Because the same amount of effort to cut calories—whether through willpower, drugs, or surgery—is met with growing resistance as ongoing weight loss increasingly activates our feedback control circuit, stimulating our appetite. In the case of the GLP-1 drugs, the weight loss caused by the initial drop in appetite is undercut by an apparent exponential increase in caloric intake as our body fights back and ratchets up our hunger again. Within 12 months, this resistance, combined with the decreased caloric needs from being lighter, matches the persistent effort to cut calories, and weight loss plateaus.[77]

Let's put some numbers on it using a validated mathematical model.

After ramping up to a full dose of semaglutide, people appear to eat nearly a thousand fewer calories a day. No wonder they initially lose so much weight. Then, their bodies push back and resist the strong GLP-1 signaling by amping up their appetites once again. But not all the way up, because they are still injecting the drugs every week. So, eventually, they end up eating only about 400 fewer calories a day.

Shouldn't they still be losing weight, though? That's still 400 fewer calories than before they started down this path. Weight loss stalls because, at that point, they are expending 400 fewer calories a day simply because they don't have to carry that extra 30 or so pounds on their body. So, with calories-in matching calories-out, weight loss stops.[78]

After You Quit

Maintaining a stable weight only lasts as long as the 400-calorie deficit continues. As soon as we stop taking the drugs, our full appetite resumes and we start regaining the weight we initially lost. Here are the two weight regain curves published in the respective drug inserts of semaglutide[79] and tirzepatide:[80]

Regained Weight Curves

Semaglutide

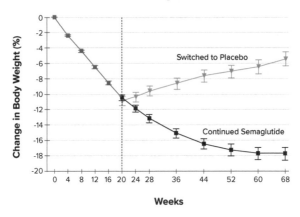

Tirzepatide

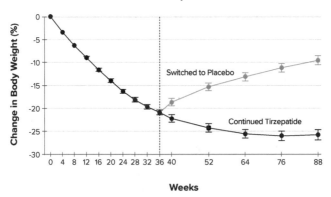

Figure 3

Rubino D, Abrahamsson N, Davies M, et al. Effect of continued weekly subcutaneous semaglutide vs placebo on weight loss maintenance in adults with overweight or obesity: the STEP 4 randomized clinical trial. *JAMA.* 2021;325(14):1414–25.

Aronne LJ, Sattar N, Horn DB, et al. Continued treatment with tirzepatide for maintenance of weight reduction in adults with obesity: the SURMOUNT-4 randomized clinical trial. *JAMA.* 2024;331(1):38–48.

All the study participants were initially started on the drugs and, on average, began losing weight. Then, some were randomized to be switched unknowingly to placebo injections. Those who continued taking the drug continued to lose weight until reaching the plateau, whereas those who switched to placebo started to regain all the weight they had initially lost.[81]

As the weight loss evaporates, so too do the benefits. In the semaglutide trial, blood pressures came down with the numbers on the scale, but then they climbed right back as if the study participants had never started the drug. In fact, blood pressures rose back to baseline even before all the weight was regained. Blood sugars and markers of systemic inflammation also started to creep back up.[82] So, we may start out obese, end up obese, and have to keep taking these drugs every day or every week for the rest of our life to hold our ground. These are considered forever drugs, the pharmaceutical industry's golden goose.[83] They're drugs for lifestyle diseases that may have to be taken lifelong because they aren't treating the underlying cause.

QUITTING BEFORE EVEN STARTING

GLP-1 drugs aren't magic bullets. Their weight-loss benefits are described as "notable but nonetheless limited."[84] The best of them can induce a weight loss of 20 to 25 percent before stalling out, and that can still leave users obese, only modestly less so. And, of course, the drugs are only effective as long as they're used,[85] yet most people stop taking them within months before they even reach an effective dose.[86]

The manufacturers recommend ramping up usage over four[87] or five months,[88] but based on more than 169,000 real-world patients using GLP-1 drugs for weight management, most individuals don't stay on their prescribed treatment for even three months, which suggests it's unlikely they're achieving any clinically meaningful weight loss. In fact, only about half appear to take the drug for *two months*, and 80 percent quit by six months.[89]

A Belly for an Arm and a Leg

Why don't people stick with it? One reason may be the cost. For instance, Wegovy, the high-dose Ozempic used for weight loss, costs up to $1,350 a month,[90] which, again, may have to be paid in perpetuity since any lost weight can pile back on if you stop taking it.[91] So, that could cost more than $16,000 a year if paid out-of-pocket for those whose insurance doesn't cover it.[92] And some say healthy eating is expensive? We could have Food Is Medicine grocery programs deliver healthy food to our door for ten times less. We could even have fully prepared meals delivered directly at a fraction of the cost of the drug.[93]

These drugs should eventually get cheaper, though. Competition will lower prices, but each of these GLP-1 drugs is protected by about 20 patents, and many until 2040 or beyond, so prices won't fall any time soon[94] in the United States (unless the U.S. government is willing to negotiate lower prices).[95]

Isn't obesity itself expensive? Yes, but even after factoring in discounted prescription prices and any reduced healthcare costs that may be achieved, these medications are not considered cost-effective. One analysis calculated that total annual healthcare expenditures *doubled* for those on these drugs from approximately $13,000 per person before starting the drug to $26,000 after. The benefits of weight loss accrue over time, but since the pounds return once drug treatment is stopped, it's understandable why insurance companies are hesitant to pay out all that money if most people are going to just stop taking it and regain the weight.[96]

Since individuals using these drugs may still end up obese when their weight loss stalls, you can imagine how it may not be worth paying a thousand dollars a month to just stay less obese. You can see why people might just cut their losses even if they lose their losses. But cost isn't the only reason so few people stay on GLP-1 drugs. In fact, the study on 169,000 users that found that most quit within a few months was a study of insured individuals who had their drug costs covered by insurance.[97] So, the main reason most people quit so soon after starting may not be due to their cost, but rather their "brutal"[98] side effects.

Why So Expensive?

Why are the drugs so costly in the first place? According to U.S. Senate Health Committee Chair Bernie Sanders, "There is no rational reason, other than greed," noting that Canadians paid $155 a month and Germans just $59 for the same drugs.[99] Danish drugmaker Novo Nordisk, maker of Ozempic and Wegovy, lists the high-dose version used for weight loss for $1,349 per month in the United States but only $92 in the United Kingdom.[100] When researchers calculated the "estimated minimum price," how much it could be manufactured and sold profitably for, they settled on $40 a month. Novo Nordisk could manufacture and distribute Wegovy for $40 a month and still earn a 10 percent

continued

profit margin.[101] But why make 10 percent profit when you can profit by more than 3,000 percent?

But don't drug companies need massive profit margins to recoup research and development costs? Developing drugs is expensive, yet, in reality, most big drug manufacturers spend more on "self-enrichment" than actual research. Novo Nordisk, for example, reportedly spends twice as much money ($7 billion) enriching its shareholders with practices such as stock buybacks to elevate stock prices than it does on all R&D ($3.4 billion).[102] Pharmaceutical companies may even spend far more on marketing drugs than developing them.[103]

While some patients were paying a thousand dollars a month for its drugs, Novo Nordisk was spending millions of dollars on meals and travel, wining and dining doctors to encourage them to prescribe them.[104] Novo Nordisk was actually suspended from a pharmaceutical industry trade association for failing to disclose its sponsorship of a training course for healthcare professionals that just so happened to plug one of its GLP-1 drugs.[105] The violation was considered egregious enough that the Royal College of Physicians severed its ties with the drug giant.[106]

COMMON GLP-1 DRUG
SIDE EFFECTS

More than half of people prescribed GLP-1 drugs stop taking them in a matter of months,[107] but older weight-loss drugs had a 98 percent failure rate.[108] And, although most people taking these types of GLP-1 mimics start out obese and end up obese no matter how long they're on them, that's just on average. A small fraction, about 1 in 25 individuals, plateaued down at an ideal weight. One person in 25 might not seem like a lot, but individuals who are obese rarely achieve an ideal weight.[109] Without something drastic like bariatric surgery, only 1 in 210 men with class 1 obesity (a BMI of 30 to 34.9) or 1 in 124 women is able to find their way back to an ideal weight.[110] So, these GLP-1 drugs really can have a dramatic effect for a select few, provided they are able to stay on them indefinitely to maintain that weight loss.[111] Even for those who can afford the cost, though, most stop taking GLP-1 drugs and the main reason is the gastrointestinal side effects.[112]

The most common side effects of Ozempic-type drugs include nausea, vomiting, diarrhea, and constipation.[113] These adverse gastrointestinal effects have been demonstrated in virtually every trial,[114] though they weren't bad enough to cause more than 15 percent of study participants to drop out, and the vast majority of adverse effects got better after they stopped taking the drugs.[115] On high-dose Ozempic, 44 percent experienced nausea, 30 percent diarrhea, 24 percent vomiting, 24 percent constipation, and 20 percent abdominal pain,[116] but 16 percent of people on *placebo* injections also experienced nausea or diarrhea. And, on placebo, 10 or 11 percent reported constipation or abdominal pain, so only about half of those side effects were due to the drugs. People don't tend to just spontaneously vomit (only 6 percent did in the placebo group), so that's more likely to be a drug-induced effect.[117]

Controlling GI Side Effects

Some people may not experience such symptoms at all, and there are steps one can take to minimize the gastrointestinal distress. The symptoms appear to be dose-dependent and tend to dissipate over time, so prescribers are encouraged to start low and go slow, gradually nudging up the dose over many months as tolerated.[118] Patients can also help stave off symptoms by eating slowly; having smaller portions; eating a low-fat diet; taking small sips of fluid; getting some fresh air; and having crackers, apples, mint, and ginger when they feel nauseated. Patients are also advised to stay hydrated, but avoid sports drinks, dairy products, coffee, alcohol, and soft drinks. Those with unusually severe symptoms may want to try avoiding all drinks during meals. However, if symptoms persist or worsen, immediately notify your healthcare provider.[119]

Doctors can also prescribe anti-vomiting drugs to counter the side effects of the weight-loss drugs,[120] but will we still lose weight if we don't feel nauseated all the time? Yes, even people who don't feel sick to their stomach can experience the appetite suppression induced by the drugs that leads to weight loss.[121]

Stop the Drugs Well Before Elective Surgery

GLP-1 makes us feel fuller for longer by slowing down the rate at which food leaves our stomach. That contributes to the nausea and vomiting. It can also lead to a serious complication if we have to go under anesthesia for surgery.[122]

GLP-1 drugs so slow the emptying of the stomach that the American Society of Anesthesiologists recommends that people stop taking the drugs for up to a week prior to procedures. The fear is we'll have a full stomach—even if we've been fasting for eight or more hours—and aspirate contents into our lungs while on the operating table. However, a week off the drugs may not be enough.[123]

Despite fasting, patients taking these drugs had a higher prevalence of increased residual stomach contents, even when they stopped taking the drugs seven days before anesthesia.[124] So, prior to elective surgery, consider stopping a drug like Ozempic at least *three weeks* before the procedure.[125]

Stopping these drugs for a month or so may not be tenable for those with diabetes, however, as they need them to control their blood sugars. But if you're taking them solely for weight loss, it's a good idea to skip a few weekly doses if you know you're going in for surgery.[126]

Controlling Muscle Loss Side Effects

Ozempic and other GLP-1 drugs may undoubtedly help people lose weight; however, the *type* of weight that is lost is often overlooked.[127]

Typically, when people who are obese lose weight, about 25 percent of their total weight loss is fat-free mass—meaning essentially their *lean* mass, including their muscles. So, of every four pounds lost on the scale, one of those pounds isn't fat.[128] But, on drugs like Ozempic, as much as *40 percent* of the total weight lost is lean mass.[129] Researchers found that those on high-dose Ozempic or tirzepatide lost about 14 pounds of lean mass, about one-eighth of all the lean mass in their body.[130] To help put that in perspective, that's worse than the amount of lean mass lost by people with malignancies like esophageal cancer that cause them to waste away.[131]

Those paid by the companies making these weight-loss drugs have questioned whether the amount of muscle mass lost is "clinically relevant."[132] Considering that the drugs cause the loss of lean mass "comparable to a decade or more of aging," I would say so.[133] Nevertheless, drug industry consultants argue that even if 40 percent of the weight lost is in fact lean mass, the majority (60 percent) is fat, so people still achieve a better lean-to-fat ratio in the end.[134] But that's only on the first go-around. Remember, most people don't stick to these drugs for more than a few months because of the cost, side effects, or even drug shortages.[135] And when the pounds of body fat return, there's a concern that the pounds of lost muscle mass may *not*, so users may end up with more fat in the end.[136]

This kind of weight cycling has been associated with extra fat deposition on the body, especially around the abdomen and waist. Using MRI imaging, the gold-standard method, to directly visualize muscle mass, researchers found that the more times people cycle their weight, the more their body composition appears to worsen.[137] The "profound level" of lean mass loss associated with GLP-1 weight-loss drugs would be expected to increase the risk of frailty, though this concern remains theoretical since such outcomes have yet to be studied.[138]

The good news is there's something we can do about this. Engaging in exercise, especially resistance exercises like strength training, can cut the proportion of fat-free mass that is lost by 50 percent or more.[139] As you can see in figure 4 below, based on half a dozen studies of caloric restriction for weight loss, researchers found that those in *non*-exercising groups lost *more* weight than those in the group with the same caloric restriction plus resistance exercise. This might seem counter-intuitive, until you consider what kind of weight was being lost. Without the resistance exercise, the study participants lost more lean mass, whereas those who were exercising apparently didn't lose any.[140,141]

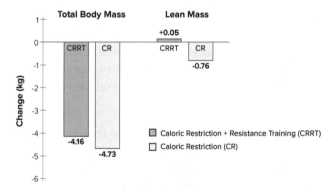

Effects of Caloric Restriction and Resistance Training vs. Caloric-Restriction Alone on Body Composition

Figure 4

Sardeli AV, Komatsu TR, Mori MA, Gaspari AF, Chacon-Mikahil MPT. Resistance training prevents muscle loss induced by caloric restriction in obese elderly individuals: a systematic review and metaanalysis. *Nutrients* 2018;10:423

Resistance exercise is considered an effective approach to at least mitigate the loss of muscle mass associated with weight loss. Those starting GLP-1 drugs are encouraged to start a tailored resistance training "without delay."[142]

Ozempic Face

"Ozempic face" is a term that whipped up a media frenzy, used to describe a distorted facial appearance among users of the drug.[143] (Similar accounts have been made of "Ozempic butt."[144]) Media reports have linked the drug with facial aging, but the sagging appearance has been ascribed simply to the accelerated loss of fat in the face.[145] While this interpretation seems logical, a review of the phenomenon concluded that "this explanation cannot fully account for the markedly accelerated facial aging...." Other factors suspected as being responsible for the appearance of premature facial aging include the loss of facial muscle mass, diminished structural integrity of the skin, and changes in stem cell function and hormonal secretion.[146]

Gallbladder issues are another side effect of rapid weight loss by any means. Excess cholesterol shed from fat cells can crystalize in our bile like rock candy, forming gallstones.[147] In a way, though, both the loss of muscle and the gain of gallstones may just be signs of how effective these drugs can be for losing weight.[148] However, as the popularity of these drugs soars, rare but serious adverse effects are emerging.[149]

MORE SERIOUS GLP-1 DRUG SIDE EFFECTS

The package inserts for both GLP-1 weight-loss drugs, semaglutide and tirzepatide, list a series of "warnings and precautions" that include thyroid tumors, acute inflammation of the pancreas (pancreatitis), acute gallbladder disease, acute kidney injury (that may stem from dehydration due to excess vomiting or diarrhea[150]), allergic reactions, a heightened risk of bottoming out blood sugars while on blood sugar–lowering medications, worsening eye disease for those with type 2 diabetes, an increase in heart rate requiring monitoring, and suicidal thoughts and behaviors.[151,152]

Suicide

Let's start with the good news. While adverse psychiatric events are biologically plausible since GLP-1 receptors are expressed throughout the brain, a meta-analysis of randomized controlled trials did not highlight any detrimental effects of GLP-1 drugs on mental health, including suicide.[153] Those suffering with mental illnesses are typically excluded from clinical trials, though, so the findings may have limited relevance. However, newer studies conducted out in the real world outside of a research setting similarly found no clear increased risk of suicidal thoughts and behaviors.[154] One study of hundreds of thousands of overweight individuals on anti-obesity drugs even found that those on semaglutide had less than half the risk of suicidal thoughts compared to those on older weight-loss drugs.[155] You could imagine how the improved efficacy of the new GLP-1 drugs could help elevate mood.

Thyroid Cancer

What about cancer? Both semaglutide and tirzepatide carry a so-called black box warning for thyroid cancer risk. This is the FDA's strictest caution about potentially life-threatening hazards. In rodents, these drugs cause thyroid tumors that are dose-dependent and duration-dependent at clinically relevant exposures, meaning the types of doses prescribed to humans. We don't know yet whether these weight-loss drugs cause a similar type of cancer in people. To be on the safe side, the drugs shouldn't be prescribed for high-risk individuals, such as those with a personal or family history of thyroid cancer. (Not that the rats had thyroid cancer running in their families.) Doctors should also counsel their patients to remain alert to thyroid tumor symptoms, including a lump or swelling in the neck, trouble swallowing, shortness of breath, or persistent hoarseness. The value of screening users for thyroid tumors with ultrasound is considered uncertain, since no such studies have been done.

The first major human study that raised concern about the risk of thyroid cancer in humans was published in 2023.[156] Researchers found a significantly increased risk of thyroid cancer in individuals using these drugs, particularly after taking them for a few years. Could their findings have just been a fluke? Unfortunately, after putting together all the best studies, a systematic review and meta-analysis of randomized controlled trials also found a significant increase in the risk, approximately 50 percent greater odds of thyroid cancer.[157] That sounds worse than it is, though, since thyroid cancer is so rare overall.

The incidence of thyroid cancer in this kind of population is 0.285 cases per 1,000 patient years. That means, over a span of ten years, we would only expect about three people out of a thousand to get that particular cancer.[158] So, even if risk is bumped up by 50 percent, we're still only talking about four in a thousand getting thyroid cancer over a decade, compared to three in a thousand, had they not started taking the GLP-1 drugs. That translates to a five-year "number needed to harm" of 1,349. So, even if this were truly cause and effect, 1,349 people would need to take the drugs for five years to cause a single additional case of thyroid cancer.

And even if you are the unlucky soul who gets it, thyroid cancer is fairly mild as cancers go. The relative five-year survival rate—the likelihood you'll be alive five years after diagnosis, compared to people without the cancer—is 98.4 percent.[159] The same cannot be said for pancreatic cancer, which has a relative five-year survival rate of only 12.8 percent. Almost everyone diagnosed with pancreatic cancer is killed by it.[160]

Pancreatic Cancer

An analysis of the prescription records of 16 million Americans found that the use of GLP-1 drugs like Ozempic was associated with nine times more pancreatitis and four times the risk of bowel obstruction, compared to taking an older class of weight-loss drugs.[161] The slowing of our digestive tract[162] is partly responsible for both the pros (feeling fuller for longer) and cons (vomiting and feeling nauseated) of GLP-1 drugs, but sometimes our gut can become so sluggish that it stops working and results in an intestinal blockage.[163] Bowel obstructions can become a surgical emergency, but their occurrence is rare. The number needed to harm after one year of drug use is 1,223, meaning more than a thousand people would have to take the drug for a year to cause a single extra bowel obstruction. So, even after ten years of taking the GLP-1 drugs, our cumulative risk would be less than 1 percent.[164]

What about the 800 percent increased risk of pancreatitis?[165] Digestive hormones like GLP-1 have multiple effects on multiple organs, perhaps more "magic shotgun" than "magic bullet," but maybe not so magical for the pancreas.[166] GLP-1 receptors are expressed abundantly throughout our pancreas, and, in response to GLP-1 drugs, cells in our pancreas proliferate, swelling the organ and potentially squeezing off ducts.[167] This can cause pancreatitis, at least in rats. Human studies that followed suggest that GLP-1 drugs may increase the odds of pancreatitis as much as sixfold.[168]

Pancreatitis is not the primary concern, though.[169] Acute pancreatitis can be acutely painful, but the major worry involves "subclinical" (asymptomatic) inflammation of the pancreas that can lead to pancreatic cancer.[170] The pro-proliferative actions of GLP-1 might accelerate the progression of potentially premalignant changes found in the pancreases of the exposed rats towards cancer.[171]

Remember how these GLP-1 drugs were modeled off a compound found in the saliva of the Gila monster?[172] Few have paused to ponder why a desert lizard would produce such a thing. The Gila monster goes for weeks or even months without eating and conserves energy between meals by shrinking its digestive tract, including its pancreas. So, when it finally does eat again, it needs a way to rapidly proliferate its tissues.[173]

A *British Medical Journal* (*BMJ*) investigation reviewed thousands of pages of documents obtained through freedom of information requests and "unearthed unpublished data from animal and human studies that point to pathological changes in the pancreas," as well as "attempts by drug companies to suppress scientific debate through pressure on academics and medical journals."[174] Why was important safety data withheld from the public?[175] A *BMJ* editorial cites the "three monkey paradigm":

> *"Companies are legally responsible for monitoring the safety of their own products, but self evidently cannot be held responsible for tackling a safety concern that does not exist. A concern that can be plausibly doubted or denied carries no legal liability, whereas one that gives rise to serious consideration (even in internal emails, which are discoverable) leaves the door wide open to litigation. Inviting companies to monitor the safety of their own products thus provides them with the strongest possible incentive for failing to do so, an instance of the law of unintended consequences. The three monkeys, who neither hear nor see nor speak, have been allowed to flourish at the heart of our system for protecting the public."*[176]

"After careful reflection," wrote a professor of medicine at the esteemed Mayo Clinic, "most patients and clinicians may opt to avoid GLP-1 based drugs or at least avoid using them...for a prolonged period of time."[177]

Those pointed statements were made before a pivotal human study confirmed these fears. Researchers obtained high-quality, transplant-grade pancreases from brain-dead organ donors who had been taking GLP-1 drugs for at least a year before they died and found that every pancreas showed abnormalities, including marked enlargement, dysplasia, or even a few small tumors.[178]

Thousands of pancreatic cancer cases have been reportedly tied to GLP-1 drugs, like Ozempic, based on the FDA's Adverse Events Reporting System,[179] but such databases that rely on voluntary reporting are limited by the potential for reporting bias.[180] Consider the Centers for Disease Control and Prevention's Vaccine Adverse Events Reporting System (VAERS) database. Researchers found that the more states were inclined to vote Republican, the more likely adverse reactions from COVID-19 vaccines were submitted.[181] Might there be a similar reporting bias among those who submit their pancreatic cancer to the FDA? It remains unclear whether the use of GLP-1 drugs is linked to pancreatic cancer,[182] and it may be years before we definitively know one way or the other. "The fundamental question," asked one Johns Hopkins University drug safety researcher, "is who bears the burden of the passage of time while these debates are settled?"[183]

But, if you *really* don't want to get cancer, then you really don't want to be at an unhealthy weight. Based on a study following millions of people, researchers found that the longer we're overweight or obese, the higher our apparent risk of 18 different types of cancer.[184] So, even if these drugs cause thyroid and pancreatic cancers, might these drugs actually lower our *overall* cancer risk if they result in enough weight loss? A meta-analysis of bariatric surgery studies found that those going under the knife tend to lose so much weight that they have a significantly lower risk of getting cancer and appear to cut their risk of dying from cancer nearly in half.[185] Based on these sorts of data, a modelling study suggests that widespread usage of GLP-1 weight-loss drugs could prevent more than one out of a hundred cancers over the next 25 years[186]—and cancer is just the United States' second leading killer.[187] Wouldn't the cardiovascular benefits of losing a lot of weight alone outweigh any potential risks?[188]

THE RISKS OF GLP-1 DRUGS VS. THE RISKS OF OBESITY

The absolute risks for serious side effects like pancreatitis, thyroid cancer, and bowel obstruction are about 1 percent or less per year of using GLP-1-type drugs.[189] Of course, when millions of individuals are taking them, even relatively rare side effects will occur in a large number of people, but obesity itself has serious side effects.

Ironically, one potential side effect of GLP-1 drugs is that they can be too effective. They can suppress the appetite so much that there are case reports of excessive weight loss, for example, individuals going on diets "comprised only of water and diet soda" or starting an eat-once-a-week diet.[190] Choosing to starve is hardly healthy, but any discussion of the pros and cons of these drugs must take into account the benefits of losing excess weight.

Choosing Surgery

Excess body fat is a major risk factor for metabolic diseases involving nearly every organ of our body, such as type 2 diabetes, heart disease, stroke, dementia, liver disease, sleep apnea, osteoarthritis, infertility, and several cancers, including breast cancer and colon cancer. For some, surgery may seem like their best or only choice.

Liposuction currently reigns as the most popular cosmetic surgery in the world, and its effects are indeed only cosmetic.[191] A study published in *The New England Journal of Medicine* assessed 15 obese women before and after having about 20 pounds of fat sucked out of their bodies, resulting in nearly a 20 percent drop in their total body fat.[192] Normally, if we lose even just 5 to 10 percent of our body weight in fat, we get significant improvements in blood pressure, blood sugars, inflammation, cholesterol, and triglycerides,[193] but none of those benefits materialized after the massive liposuction.[194]

This suggests subcutaneous fat, the fat under our skin, is not the problem. The metabolic insults of obesity arise from the *visceral* fat surrounding or even infiltrating our inner organs, like the fat marbling our muscles and livers. The way we lose that fat, the dangerous fat, is to take in fewer calories than we burn, which can be accomplished through appetite-suppressing drugs or surgical rearrangement of our anatomy, for example.

The use of bariatric surgery has exploded from about 40,000 procedures per year, as noted in the first international survey in 1998,[195] to hundreds of thousands now performed each year in the United States alone.[196] How can the overall outcomes of bariatric surgery inform our discussion of the overall outcomes of GLP-1 drugs?

Health Outcomes of Bariatric Surgery

Bariatric surgery is not exactly a benign procedure.[197] Roux-en-Y gastric bypass, one of the most popular techniques, is considered the "'gold standard' method given its safety, with a mortality rate < 0.5 %." (It's jarring to hear boasting about not killing more than 1 in 200 people in the operating room.) The procedure involves major surgery but can induce a long-term weight loss of about 25 percent, which rivals some of the best results of the new GLP-1 drugs.[198] So, if you only care about living longer, might the benefits of weight loss outweigh the risks of dying on the operating table?

A meta-analysis based on millions of patients found that only about 1 in 1,250 people is killed by the surgery. Since the ones who don't lose their lives tend to lose so much weight, even taking perioperative mortality into account, bariatric surgery has been associated with a six-year-longer lifespan.[199] In this way, choosing a surgical intervention may significantly extend our life, on average, even after taking into account the risk of dying from the procedure.

Bariatric surgery does carry a relatively high risk of complications, though. In the first five years after the surgery, approximately one in four patients experiences adverse effects, and, for one in 50, it's so bad they have to get back onto the operating table for surgical revision.[200] That's one advantage of the drug approach. If you experience a serious side effect, it may go away when you stop taking the drug, but if you've already had most of your stomach removed or your intestines rearranged, there may be less that can be done.

Researchers looked at the impact of bariatric surgery on more than five dozen health outcomes, and although people who underwent surgery may be more likely to kill themselves, break bones, and suffer acid reflux, they also appear to be less likely to get and die from cancer, diabetes, and cardiovascular disease. Of the 66 statistically significant health outcome findings, 85 percent showed an apparent protective effect of bariatric surgery, including the risk of dying from all causes put together.[201]

So, generally, the benefits of bariatric surgery far outweigh the risks, but that says less about the benefits of the procedure and more about the risks of carrying excess body fat. With the GLP-1 drugs, we see largely similar improvements in risk factors, like blood sugar control, blood pressure, and cholesterol,[202] but the risk-versus-benefit balance really depends on clinical disease outcomes. Do people really live longer on these drugs? Have fewer heart attacks?

Health Outcomes of GLP-1 Drugs

"Thinner is better" is the conventional wisdom when it comes to minimizing the risk of cardiovascular events, like heart attacks and strokes.[203] However, there have been cases in which past weight-loss medications led to *increased* cardiovascular risk despite significant reductions in body fat.[204] So we can't just assume that drug-induced weight loss will always help our heart. If GLP-1 drugs like Ozempic could reduce cardiovascular events, that would significantly tip the scales in their favor, as heart attacks and strokes are among our leading causes of death.[205] Physicians have been prescribing GLP-1 drugs for nearly 20 years to patients with diabetes. What do the studies show?

Some trials have found that, among high-risk individuals with diabetes, risk of cardiovascular events was significantly lower for those randomized to Ozempic, compared to placebo, but other trials did not. Drug company-funded researchers spun the lack of benefit as a positive, describing the cardiovascular risk as "not inferior to that of placebo."[206] It was considered a relief that it wasn't worse than placebo, since so many weight-loss drugs had caused problems in the past. No effect on cardiovascular risk is better than increasing it.

Enough evidence of benefit did accrue, though, so Ozempic was approved for cardioprotection among high-risk individuals with type 2 diabetes in 2020.[207,208] But maybe the reduction in cardiovascular risk was just due to the lowering of blood sugars rather than the lowering of body weight. From an obesity medication standpoint, the question is: What about cardiovascular outcomes for people *without* diabetes?

Researchers found that, in patients with preexisting cardiovascular disease who are overweight or obese, but do not have diabetes, those randomized to weight-loss doses of Ozempic had an overall lower rate of having a cardiovascular event like a heart attack or stroke or dying from it, compared to placebo. That's promising, but note the caveat: The researchers only considered individuals with *preexisting* cardiovascular disease.[209] The effects of these weight-loss drugs on the prevention of cardiovascular events in those without diagnosed atherosclerotic disease have not yet been determined.

Still, a lot of people carrying excess weight have a history of heart attack, stroke, or peripheral vascular disease. How meaningful was the afforded protection? Over a period of a few years, 8 percent of individuals with cardiovascular disease suffered another event on the placebo, but only 6.5 percent suffered a subsequent cardiovascular event on the drug. Going from 8 to 6.5 is a 20 percent drop.[210] Unfortunately, many news stories focused on that 20 percent *relative* risk reduction rather than on the *absolute* risk reduction of just 1.5 percent. Yes, 8 to 6.5 is a 20 percent drop, but, at the same time, we're only reducing our *absolute* risk by 1.5 percent. In other words, 67 people would have to take the drug for a few years to prevent a single heart attack, stroke, or cardiovascular death.[211] That may not sound like much on an individual scale. What are the odds you're going to be that one in sixty-seventh person? But, on a population scale, it's tremendous. In fact, it's right up there with cholesterol-lowering statin drugs, which have an absolute risk reduction in the same 1.5 percent ballpark.[212] So, in March 2024, the FDA approved high-dose Ozempic for use beyond weight loss and also authorized its use for reducing cardiovascular risk in those with preexisting cardiovascular disease.[213]

Do GLP-1 Drug Benefits Outweigh Their Harms?

Among those with pre-existing cardiovascular disease, the benefits would be expected to far outweigh the known risks. What about everyone else? In the summer of 2024, the first quantitative benefit-versus-harm balance analysis was published. The researchers concluded that those achieving a 10 percent weight loss had a more than 90 percent chance that the benefits of taking the drugs outweigh the harms, but the opposite was found for individuals achieving only a 5 percent weight loss.[214]

Here's how the researchers broke it down: If 1,000 people go on these GLP-1 drugs for two years, 375 of them would be expected to lose at least 10 percent of their body weight and gain all the ancillary benefits that weight loss would bring. On the other side of the equation, 221 people would suffer from nausea, 118 from constipation, 110 from vomiting, 100 from diarrhea, 84 from an upset stomach, 57 from hair loss, 51 from excessive farting, 46 from excessive burping, 43 from upper abdominal pain, 41 people from lower abdominal pain, 22 from dizziness, 17 from low blood sugars, 13 from headaches, 8 from gallstones, 4 from reactions at the injection site, and 4 would suffer from pancreatitis.[215]

Of course, the net benefit-versus-harm calculation would be highly dependent on different people's willingness to accept different harms. For example, someone who's already bald won't be concerned about hair loss. The analysis also doesn't take into account that the benefits peter out. As previously discussed, weight loss stalls after about a year on the drugs, but their harms may continue. So, once we've plateaued and stop losing weight, do we stop taking the drug and lose any benefits as the weight comes back, or do we keep taking it to maintain the initial weight loss (even though we get no further weight-loss benefits) while the potential for harms continues to accumulate?

At this time, we don't know about the long-term harms or benefits because some of these drugs and dosing schedules are so new. To complicate matters, the American Academy of Pediatrics has suggested offering these drugs for teens and even tweens as young as age 12.[216] These drugs work by acting on the brain, so who knows what effect they might have on childhood development and beyond if young people end up taking them for the rest of their lives.[217]

In the end, it's a familiar story, concluded a critical analysis of GLP-1 drugs in the journal of the American Diabetes Association: "A new class of antidiabetic agents is rushed to market and widely promoted in the absence of any evidence of long-term beneficial outcomes. Evidence of harm accumulates, but is vigorously discounted...The manufacturers are expected—quite unrealistically—to monitor the safety of their own product. We should be thankful that those responsible for aircraft safety do not operate on the same assumption...."[218]

Although we now have evidence of *near*-term benefit over a few years, we cannot assume long-term safety until it has been demonstrated.[219]

Compounding the Issue

The discussion of risk versus benefit is moot if we aren't taking the actual drug. Shortage of these medications has led patients to compounding pharmacies that offer versions of the drugs that have not been approved by the FDA.[220] In the past, compounding pharmacies have been plagued with serious safety issues, like an epidemic of fungal meningitis caused by moldy bottles of drugs. In that instance, 751 patients were ultimately affected and more than 60 patients died.[221]

At least compounding pharmacies are regulated at the state level.[222] Consumer protections may be missing entirely at so-called medical spas and "wellness clinics" that may inject people with who-knows what. People don't seem to be paying much attention to repeated FDA warnings[223,224] about compounded GLP-1 drugs, though. As the title of a *Rolling Stone* article put it: "The FDA Warned Ozempic Users. They Don't Give a F-ck."[225]

BOOSTING GLP-1 WITH DIET AND LIFESTYLE

Given the potential side effects of GLP-1 agonists, long-term unknowns, and cost, can we *just say no* to the drugs and get the benefits of GLP-1 without the risks by boosting it naturally with diet and lifestyle changes?

Well, there's exercise.[226] To date, there have been five studies of exercise and GLP-1, and four out of the five of them found higher concentrations of total GLP-1 after both high-intensity interval training and moderate-intensity continuous training, with no apparent difference between the two.[227] Unfortunately, there appeared to be "publication bias"; some trials that failed to show an effect may have been quietly shelved, thereby skewing the results. So, the effect of exercise on GLP-1 remains uncertain, but what's the downside of exercising? The evidence is overwhelming that nearly everyone can benefit from becoming more physically active.[228]

What about diet? A variety of natural foods, beverages, and spices has been shown to boost our own natural GLP-1 levels.[229] Enough to work as an alternative to the drugs that mimic GLP-1, like Ozempic?

Can Our Natural GLP-1 Rival GLP-1 Mimics?

Normally, the levels of GLP-1 in our bloodstream rise and fall in response to meal ingestion. On GLP-1-mimicking medications, drug levels in our blood are said to remain "relatively stable and high"—but "high" is an understatement.[230] In the two hours after we eat a meal, natural GLP-1 rises to around 20 or 30 picomoles per liter.[231] In contrast, the levels of

GLP-1-lookalike drugs typically reach around 20 to 30 *nano*moles per liter. *Pico-* means trillionth, and *nano-* means billionth. So, drug levels are a thousand times higher.[232] How could boosting natural levels even come close?

A small part of the dramatic discrepancy may be an artifact of drawing blood from people's veins to run lab tests. Since natural GLP-1 is rapidly deactivated by an enzyme in our blood, by the time GLP-1 is secreted by our gut, makes it through our liver, heart, and lungs, then out into our arteries only to later return via the veins where the lab tech draws our blood, the levels seen are lower than the *arterial* levels that GLP-1 receptors are exposed to throughout our body.[233]

The more consequential difference between natural GLP-1 levels and those of the drug have to do with the amount that's free-floating in the blood. After all, how do drugs like Ozempic stay in our body for weeks instead of the minutes natural GLP-1 does?[234] The drugs are chemically modified to stick to the most abundant protein in our blood. So, even though the total drug level in our blood is in the nanomolar range, it's so tightly bound to protein that the *active* level in our blood—the amount that's free to interact with tissue receptors—is around a hundred times less, which means at least down in the picomolar range. Thus, although drug levels would seem to far exceed normal levels of GLP-1 at first glance, they may actually approach that of GLP-1 after strong natural stimulation.[235] The primary action of appetite reduction happens in the brain, though, which may not depend on blood levels.[236]

The primary source of GLP-1 secretion in the body is the gut, but the regulation of food intake by GLP-1 occurs in the brain.[237] GLP-1 can cross the blood-brain barrier,[238] but wouldn't it get eaten up by enzymes in our blood before much of it even made it up there? There are nerves in our brainstem that can also secrete GLP-1, and there's a direct connection between our gut and our brainstem called the *vagus nerve*. The thought is that GLP-1 produced in our gut in response to a meal stimulates our vagus nerve to convey this signal to our brain, bypassing any need for direct blood transport.[239] In that case, why do we have GLP-1 receptors on organs throughout our body[240]—including our pancreas, kidneys, liver, and heart—if the hormone acts mainly through the vagus nerve? It's possible that strong dietary stimuli can boost levels in the blood high enough to also activate these peripheral receptors.

Normally after a meal, GLP-1 may work by sending an appetite-reducing signal to our brain directly through the vagus nerve. Our brain then relays the message to the relevant systems throughout our body. High levels of a GLP-1 mimic like Ozempic in the blood can circulate directly through the bloodstream to all those organs, including the brain.[241] Might a strong dietary GLP-1 stimulus be able to do both—trigger appetite-reducing signals through the vagus nerve and also activate GLP-1 receptors on peripheral organs?

When different levels of the GLP-1 hormone are dripped straight into people's veins, a dose-dependent reduction in both hunger and food intake can be observed.[242] However, the dosages used in infusion studies elevated baseline levels fourfold or more, whereas the bump in blood levels from food tended to only double them.[243] So, while high-dose GLP-1 infusion drives a clear change in hunger and eating behavior, there has been skepticism that inducing GLP-1 secretion through diet would have a measurable effect.[244] But we now have research showing these effects can be achieved at diet-relevant levels.

If you recall, food naturally boosts blood levels of GLP-1 up around 20 picomoles per liter. Research has found that simply elevating our GLP-1 levels to 15, 10, or even just 5 picomoles per liter can result in a significant drop in food intake—like eating 30 to 35 percent less of an all-you-can-eat meal.[245] This is well within doable dietary ranges.

So, even a slight increase in levels by dietary manipulation of GLP-1 secretion could be sufficient to have clinical relevance. We don't have to strive for levels comparable to those obtained using drugs. This makes sense. Why would our body naturally produce an appetite-suppressing hormone in response to food if it didn't end up suppressing our appetite?

Chew on This

GLP-1 secretion doesn't just depend on what we eat, but how we eat. When researchers had people eat the same meal but chew each bite either 15 times or 40 times, the levels of GLP-1 rose higher after 40 chews than 15. Additionally, those who chewed 40 times ended up consuming about 75 fewer calories than the 15-time chewers.[246] So, chewing more may help us keep our weight down, but who wants to count how many times they chew every bite they take? What if we just ate chewier foods?

Researchers had people eat shredded cabbage, which requires a lot of chewing, or the same amount of pureed cabbage, which doesn't. The same food, the same amount of food, with differences just in chewing. GLP-1 blood levels were higher for up to 90 minutes after the shredded cabbage compared to pureed.[247] The researchers were careful to make sure the participants in each group ate at the same rate, because eating slower can also result in a greater GLP-1 response.

When research subjects were asked to eat the same amount of ice cream over a period of either 5 minutes or 30 minutes, those who ate at the slower rate experienced a significant boost in GLP-1 levels in their blood for hours after having the ice cream, about a 30 percent bump overall.[248] On average, the participants were overweight, but much slimmer than the average American.[249] Would the results be the same for individuals who are obese and could really benefit from the extra GLP-1 boost?

Testing the same ice cream protocol, researchers found that teens who are obese had the same outcome as adults who are overweight (but not obese), a significantly higher GLP-1 response after slower eating. But the rate of eating didn't seem to matter in obese adults. The same was found for satiety. Obese adolescents felt fuller and more satiated for longer when they ate more slowly, but speed of eating didn't seem to matter in obese adults.[250]

At least for some, chewing more and eating more slowly may raise GLP-1 levels no matter what is consumed, but there are certain foods that specifically boost GLP-1.

FOODS THAT BOOST OUR GLP-1

A review article entitled "Boosting GLP-1 by Natural Products" concluded that "compelling" data suggest that red onions, buckwheat, ginseng, ginger root, gardenia, green tea, wheat fiber, soybeans, cinnamon, berberine (found in barberries), quercetin (in capers), curcumin (in turmeric), and resveratrol (in grapes) "each have potent effects on GLP-1 activity."[251] The hope is that increasing the release of our own GLP-1 hormone by eating specific foods could have similar benefits to those that may be achieved from GLP-1-mimicking drugs—without their potentially disabling side effects.

Any time a secondary source, like that review article, makes a statement of fact, it's always important to double-check the original studies. For example, the review cites three studies purportedly showing that soy can induce GLP-1 secretion but fails to disclose the findings were in mice,[252] rats,[253] and petri dishes.[254] The evidence cited for ginseng was also limited to rats[255] and test tubes.[256] Components derived from gardenias also purportedly "potentiate GLP-1 secretion," but, again, that was based only on cells and rodents.[257] When they were tested on humans, those in the gardenia group showed a *decrease* in GLP-1.[258]

What about resveratrol, the red wine compound found in some grapes? It worked in rats with diabetes,[259] but not humans with diabetes.[260]

Green tea is also on the list and is said to increase GLP-1 levels in actual human patients, but, in fact, the increase over placebo did not reach statistical significance.[261] Olive oil is said to induce higher GLP-1 concentrations than butter, but the cited study didn't show any significant difference.[262] That was on nondiabetic subjects, though. A similar study on individuals with diabetes did show a larger GLP-1 response, but only by about 15 percent.[263]

Online, you'll find so-called experts who claim that eating avocados can be "as effective as weight loss injections."[264] Mainstream media articles cite "nutritionists" who claim avocados work "just like the miracle weight loss jab Ozempic."[265] *Guacamozempic* may work if you're a rat,[266] but in humans, GLP-1 was found to be significantly lower after a meal with added avocado.[267]

What about berberine, dubbed "nature's Ozempic"?[268] A component of barberries, a dried fruit I've profiled as a treatment for acne,[269] berberine boosts GLP-1 secretion in rats and in petri dishes,[270] but there haven't yet been any GLP-1 studies of berberine on humans. What we care about, though, is weight loss, and there have been a number of studies on the effect of berberine and barberries on body weight. Their findings? No effect was found for berberine supplements or barberries themselves.[271]

Spices to Boost GLP-1

Fenugreek flopped, too. The herb seemed to boost GLP-1 signaling in a test tube,[272] but it didn't work for mice[273] and there have yet to be any human studies. However, some spices can legitimately boost GLP-1 in humans.

In a study out of Singapore, volunteers were served white rice with vegetable curry made with three different doses of spices. The bland control meal had no spices at all, just tomato puree with eggplant. The low-spice meal added a tablespoon of curry spices, plus onions, garlic, and ginger, and the third variation, the high-spice curry, had the same onions, garlic, and ginger, but double the spices, two tablespoons. The spices were turmeric, coriander seeds, cumin seeds, dried Indian gooseberry powder (also known as amla), cayenne pepper, cinnamon, and cloves in the ratio of 8:4:4:4:2:1:1. Researchers found that the average bump in GLP-1 blood concentration for those eating the low-spice and high-spice meals were 17 percent and 32 percent higher, respectively, compared to the bland control meal. All three meals had about the same calories and macronutrients, but the spicier dishes raised GLP-1 levels higher.[274]

But which spice was it? Ginger compounds boost GLP-1 in mice,[275] but not rats,[276] and we appear to react more like the rats—no effect.[277] For many of the other spices, there aren't even in vitro data, just *in silico*, meaning computer modeling that doesn't involve testing in a biological system.[278]

We do, however, have data on curcumin, the yellow compound found in the spice turmeric.

In a cross-over, randomized, controlled study, people were given 180 milligrams of curcumin, which is the amount found in about a single teaspoon of turmeric.[279] Fish oil supplements were also tested, but while the fish oil failed, the curcumin reduced the study volunteers' blood sugar spike after a meal, which is something GLP-1 and GLP-1-mimicking drugs can do. GLP-1 levels weren't directly measured in the study, but the researchers suggest it may be a GLP-1 effect, since curcumin stimulates GLP-1 in rodents and in cells in a petri dish.[280]

It wasn't until 2024 when we learned curcumin's effects on GLP-1 secretion in humans. Six months of curcumin supplementation led to a quadrupling of GLP-1 levels, compared to placebo, so turmeric may indeed have played a role in boosting GLP-1 in the curry study.[281] This may explain why a systematic review of dozens of randomized controlled trials found that turmeric or curcumin supplementation can lead to weight loss and a slimming of waist circumference.[282]

And cinnamon? Scandinavian researchers gave individuals rice pudding with and without 1 or 3 grams of cinnamon, which is about a third of a teaspoon or a full teaspoon, respectively. The full teaspoon of cinnamon more than doubled the GLP-1 bump from baseline, compared to the cinnamon-free control pudding. So, that's another spice that may work. Though people didn't report feeling any more satiated eating the cinnamony pudding compared to plain,[283] a pooled review of several meta-analyses of cinnamon found that 3 or more grams a day significantly reduces BMI and body weight.[284]

Cayenne pepper is the third spice found to boost GLP-1 in humans. After a single meal with about half a teaspoon of cayenne pepper, GLP-1 blood levels significantly increased within 15 minutes. As was the case with cinnamon, this did not seem to translate into greater feelings of fullness, but the researchers didn't measure subsequent food intake[285] and a meta-analysis of more than a dozen trials found that supplementation with capsaicin (the spicy component of hot peppers) indeed leads to weight loss.[286]

Bitter Herbs to Boost GLP-1

Most of the poisons humans use come from bitter plants, for example, strychnine and hemlock. At the same time, some of the most popular beverages in the world are bitter, like coffee, as are some of the healthiest foods, such as broccoli and other cruciferous vegetables.[287]

Bitter taste receptors aren't only on our tongue. They're also found throughout much of our digestive tract.[288] They exist on the very same cells lining our gut that secrete the appetite-suppressing hormone GLP-1.[289] And, what do you know? A number of bitter compounds have been shown to "potently stimulate" the release of hormones like GLP-1 in petri dishes and lab animals.[290] What about people? And what about beer? Beer is one of the most beloved bitter beverages, thanks to hops, the flowers of the hop plant used in its brewing.[291]

Records show that bitter herbs have traditionally been used in times of scarcity to reduce hunger, so researchers tested hop extracts on people undergoing a 24-hour fast and found it lowered feelings of hunger better than placebo.[292] Might that be a GLP-1 effect?

Taking a hop extract before a meal, in either immediate or delayed-release capsules, led to significantly more GLP-1 release than did a placebo. More importantly, when the study participants were given all-you-can-eat sandwiches a few hours later, they ate significantly less. They didn't report feeling significantly less hungry or more full, but they still ate about 200 fewer calories overall.[293]

The extract did make them feel nauseated, bloated, and barfy, but maybe that's just more evidence that the hops are working through GLP-1. After all, those are all common side effects of the GLP-1-mimicking drugs. But is *that* why they ate less? Apparently not, as the degree of gastrointestinal discomfort did not correlate with how much less they ate. The main reason I'd caution against hops is because of a toxic compound in them called 8-PN,[294] which may explain why beer[295] may be associated with a particularly high risk of getting[296] and dying from breast cancer.[297]

GLP-1 and Quinine in Tonic Water

What about quinine, perhaps the best-studied bitter substance in human history?[298] Extracted from the bark of the cinchona tree, quinine was not only the first effective treatment for malaria four centuries ago, but, remarkably, it remains a common and effective treatment to this day.[299] It can also stimulate GLP-1 secretion in people.[300] Quinine has also been found to reduce food intake and body weight in rats.[301] What about us?

The Benefits of Quinine to Boost GLP-1

A study entitled "Intragastric Quinine Administration Decreases Hedonic Eating…" described what happened when people were randomized to drink a chocolate milkshake with or without quinine in their stomach.[302] Anyone might drink less milkshake if they just had consumed something super bitter, but, no, the quinine was administered directly into the study participants' stomach through a tube, so it bypassed the bitter receptors in their mouth. Remember, though, there are also bitter receptors in our gut that we aren't even consciously aware of. Brain scans were performed, and the researchers concluded that being unknowingly slipped about 200 milligrams of quinine affected how much the participants felt like they wanted to eat, as well as how much they actually *did* eat, by interfering with reward brain circuits.

You don't have to lick some tree bark to get it. It's available in every grocery store in the form of tonic water. A liter of tonic water has about 60 to 70 milligrams of quinine,[303] and bitter lemon, another popular cocktail mixer, has about half that.[304] But reaching the 200-milligram dose of quinine used in the study would require drinking three quarts of tonic water. Do smaller doses work? Yes. Another research team tried giving just 18 milligrams of quinine or placebo, and then, an hour later, all-you-can-eat ham and cheese sandwiches. Sandwich intake was significantly lower after quinine intake than placebo, by about 14 percent.[305] So, based on the study, drinking a third of a liter of tonic water before a meal might reduce your caloric intake by 82 calories. But a third of a liter of tonic water has more than a *hundred* calories, so that wouldn't do you much good.[306]

Tonic water is essentially quinine-spiked sugar water. There are sugar-free varieties, but why not just go straight to the source? Researchers tried giving people about the same amount of quinine in the form of powdered cinchona bark, approximately a third of a teaspoon a day. They found that, compared to placebo, those in the powdered bark group had significantly more weight loss, significantly more *waist* lost, and slimmer hips, and their weight loss was in fat mass, with greater lean mass preservation.[307]

So, in humans, quinine may boost GLP-1, decrease hedonic hunger, lower appetite, decrease caloric intake, and decrease body fat. What are the downsides?

The Risks of Quinine to Boost GLP-1

The quinine in a third of a liter of tonic water or a third of a teaspoon of powdered cinchona bark can suppress appetite[308] and cause weight loss,[309] but at what cost? Quinine is a drug. In fact, it's one of the most common causes of severe drug-induced disorders.[310]

Even just the levels of quinine found in tonic water may cause "potentially fatal immunologically mediated hypersensitivity," which is basically a type of allergic reaction.[311] Quinine can interact with antibodies in our body to trigger autoimmune reactions[312] that can include chills, fever, a drop in blood pressure, painful bluish discoloration of the hands and feet, and clotting within our blood vessels that can kill us. It can also chew up our red blood cells leading to anemia, chew up our platelets leading to bleeding and bruising, and chew up our white blood cells leading to immune dysfunction, acute kidney injury, the dissolution of our muscles, liver toxicity, heart damage, respiratory failure, low blood sugars, and blindness.[313] It can also lead to toxic epidermal necrolysis, which can manifest as genital blistering,[314] including sloughed penile[315] or scrotal erosion.[316] Since quinine "even with only minute exposure from common beverages, can cause severe adverse reactions involving multiple organ systems,"[317] the "'moral of the story' is that a relaxing gin and tonic may be the cause of...several life-threatening diseases."[318]

Now, these are rare, idiosyncratic reactions. Just because peanuts can be life-threatening to someone with a peanut allergy doesn't mean everyone needs to avoid them. But quinine has *non*-hypersensitivity adverse effects, too. Even when quinine isn't eroding scrotums, for example, it may still be shrinking them. Researchers found quinine to be so damaging to the testicles of rats that they suggested exploring the use of quinine as a male contraceptive.[319]

Overdoses of quinine can be extremely toxic,[320] with vision loss a common outcome.[321] An overdose can leave us blind, affecting not only the retina in the back of our eye, but also our iris in the front, causing our pupils to become bizarrely oval-shaped.[322] The reason people may have quinine pills around their house is that some take them for nocturnal leg cramps.[323] The FDA concluded that this wasn't safe and banned its use for this purpose[324]—in both over-the-counter preparations and as a prescription drug—after receiving hundreds of reports of serious adverse events associated with quinine use, including 93 deaths.[325]

It's still available with a prescription as a malaria drug, though, and some doctors still prescribe it for leg cramps, but given its rare but serious allergic-type reactions and the risk of overdosing on quinine pills,[326] that's probably not a good idea.[327] Thankfully, following warnings by the FDA, use of quinine for treating muscle cramps has declined dramatically.[328]

Although it's been banned from one aisle of the drug store, it may still be available in another, in the form of tonic water.[329] Can the lower levels of the drug found in beverages still cause problems with vision? Following the identification by the Armed Forces Institute of Pathology of quinine in autopsy specimens from military pilot fatalities, research volunteers drank tonic water for two weeks, and, indeed, some visual abnormalities resulted.[330] Even transient blurring of vision can be disastrous if experienced by anyone operating heavy machinery at high speeds.[331] In fact, due to concern that tonic water consumption may have contributed to aviation accidents, pilots are forbidden to drink tonic water for 72 hours before flying.[332]

How much is too much? A 46-year-old man reported "increasing visual deterioration and difficulty with night driving" over a period of three months, during which he had been drinking a gallon (four liters) of tonic water each day—so that may be too much.[333] Another case involved a 75-year-old man whose heart arrhythmia was blamed on drinking a liter of tonic water.[334] His doctors suggested "the public is unaware of the risks associated with excessive consumption of tonic water," but how often does anyone drink a liter at a time?

The "no-untoward-effect level" in humans has been estimated at 52.5 milligrams of quinine a day, which is about a two and a half cups of tonic water a day.[335] However, based on ototoxicity, damage to our hearing, it's been suggested that we shouldn't drink much more than two cups a day. Both of these targets were based on extrapolations from animal models, though.[336] Since quinine was so commonly prescribed to treat leg cramps, why not just look at large populations of people and see if anything bad happened to those who were exposed to the drug? When researchers did just that, they found that individuals prescribed quinine seemed to have a 27 percent increased risk of acute kidney injury.[337] That's not great, but it isn't as bad as death.

Following 175,000 people for about six years, researchers found that those taking about 200 milligrams of quinine a day had a 25 percent greater risk of dying. Those getting about 300 daily milligrams had an 83 percent greater risk of dying, and those on 400 milligrams or more appeared to double their risk for death.[338] I recommend staying away from quinine.

The FDA has determined that carbonated drinks may safely contain up to 83 milligrams of quinine per liter,[339] but tonic water labels rarely disclose the amount, and some popular brands fail to even list quinine as an ingredient at all. How then do we know if our drink has quinine or not? Hold it up to a black light. If it contains quinine, it will light up with an iridescent bluish glow.[340] (Quinine is the secret ingredient in fluorescent jello shots.[341])

Plant-Based Meals vs. Meat-Based Meals

Vegetarian diets appear to offer significant benefits for weight reduction.[342] Might the appetite-suppressing hormone GLP-1 have anything to do with that?

Researchers have compared the effects of meaty meals versus plant-based ones on the induction of GLP-1. What happened, for example, when people either with or without diabetes ate a pork burger with cheese versus a plant-based burger made with couscous and oats?

Half an hour after eating the plant-based burger, those with diabetes experienced a doubling of GLP-1, compared to the meat burger.[343] The two meals were matched for calories, but not macronutrients, though. The meaty meal had more protein and fat, and fewer carbohydrates. Since different macros can affect GLP-1 differently, the difference in GLP-1 secretion may have had more to do with the macros than the meat. So, researchers then compared calorie- *and* macro-matched meals.

Study participants were randomized to eat either a tofu burger that was both calorie- and macronutrient-matched to a meat burger.[344] Again, those with diabetes had significantly higher increases in GLP-1 release after the veggie meal compared to the meaty one, but what about those without diabetes? In the earlier study, the plant-based meal boosted GLP-1 in those with diabetes, but not in those without. Was that discrepancy also due to the mismatch in macronutrients? The same matched tofu burger was pitted against a conventional meat burger, and the plant-based meal boosted GLP-1 levels as effectively in those with diabetes as it did in those without.[345]

Does the higher GLP-1 secretion translate into greater satiety? The study's title gives it away: "A Plant-Based Meal Increases Gastrointestinal Hormones and Satiety More Than an Energy- and Macronutrient-Matched Processed-Meat Meal in T2D [type 2 diabetic], Obese, and Healthy Men: A Three-Group Randomized Crossover Study." Satiety was greater in all groups after the plant-based meal, compared to the meat meal.[346]

Does the greater satiety translate into eating less? When study participants were given pasta with either plant-based ground beef or conventional ground beef at an all-you-can-eat buffet, they consumed significantly fewer calories of the pasta with the plant-based meat. Yet, despite eating less, they felt just as satisfied, full, and satiated. This was unlikely a GLP-1 effect, however, since rather than GLP-1 driving lower food intake, lower food intake appeared to drive lower GLP-1.[347]

Mycoprotein, which makes up meat substitutes like Quorn, comes from the mushroom kingdom rather than the plant kingdom.[348] Research shows that mycoprotein products are so satiating that they not only cause a decrease in intake at an all-you-can-eat meal, but also subsequent appetite suppression such that there's a decrease in caloric intake over the entire day.[349] Compared to chicken, Quorn led to an average reduction of 188 calories, but that was accomplished without altering GLP-1.

So, GLP-1 may not be the reason plant-based meals have been found to be more satiating or why whole food, plant-based diets have been shown to result in greater weight loss than any other eating pattern.[350] It may be because plant-based diets are associated with an improved gut microbiome, increased insulin sensitivity, better metabolism, and reduced calorie density.[351] Dietary fiber alone can improve our microbiome and reduce calorie density, and a few types of fiber may be able to also boost GLP-1.

Restoring Our Natural GLP-1 Satiety Circuit

L-cells are the specialized cells lining our digestive tract that produce appetite-suppressing hormones, like GLP-1. In addition to detecting certain bitter and pungent molecules, receptors on their surface respond to carbohydrates, proteins, and fats.[352] If these L-cells churn out appetite-suppressing hormones in response to carbs, proteins, and fats, why is there an obesity epidemic? Why are so many gaining so much weight?

The problem is the majority of GLP-1-producing L-cells are located at the end of our digestive tract[353]—at the end of our small intestine, known as the *distal ileum*—and especially in our colon, but most of the nutrients we digest are absorbed high up in our small intestine, closer to our mouth. Since those nutrients don't reach the distal ileum and colon where most L-cells are located,[354] a natural satiety mechanism known as the *ileal brake*[355] may rarely be activated.

Activating the Ileal Brake

The ileal brake is an intestinal feedback loop that tamps down our hunger.[356] When calories reach the ilium, the end of our small intestine, L-cells are activated and GLP-1 is produced, which puts the brakes on eating more.[357] Our appetite is dialed down, and the rate at which food leaves our stomach slows. This has been shown experimentally. When researchers inserted a nine-foot tube down study participants' throats and dripped in any calories—sugar, protein, or fat—their ileal brake was activated. When the subjects then sat down to an all-you-can-eat meal, they ate more than 100 fewer calories than those in the placebo group who had instead just gotten water dripped in their tube.[358] With the ileal brake activated, we just don't feel as hungry. We feel just as full, eating significantly less.

But, our natural GLP-1 satiety mechanism fails because most components of the food we eat are quickly digested and absorbed at the beginning of our small intestine, never making it to the end of the small intestine where our GLP-1-secreting cells are concentrated.[359] Why would our body design an appetite regulation system based on calories ending up in our colon, when most calories get absorbed much earlier in our digestive tract, no matter how much we eat?

Because when we were evolving, there was no such thing as table sugar. There was no such thing as Wonder Bread. No such thing as vegetable oil. For the millions of years before we began to sharpen spears, mill grains, or boil sugarcane, our entire physiology is presumed to have evolved in the context of eating what our great ape cousins did[360]—a diet "comprised of leaves, roots, fruits, and nuts."[361] We started using tools during the Paleolithic period, about 2 million years ago, but we and other great apes have been evolving since the Miocene era, which goes back as far as 20 million years.[362] So, for as much as the first 90 percent of our hominoid existence, our body evolved on mostly whole plant foods.[363]

Here is why that matters: The cells of plants have cellular walls that are made out of fiber, which act as an indigestible physical barrier. So, many of those calories remain trapped until the good gut bugs in our colon consume that fiber, and out spill the contents of plant cells to signal GLP-1 release. On the other hand, the cells of animals are encased in easily digestible membranes, so when we eat a steak, for example, the enzymes in our gut can more effortlessly liberate the calories. Since most of the protein, fat, and carbohydrates (like milk sugars) from animal foods get absorbed early in the small intestine, they aren't present to activate many of the satiety cells that secrete the GLP-1 hormone farther down our GI tract.[364] It's the same when we eat highly processed plant foods, like sugar water (soda), white flour, and oil.

What if we walled off our calories? That is, what if we made sure as many of our calories as possible were encased in cell walls? In other words, from whole, intact, plant foods.

The Five-Letter F-Word

Think about eating a nut. Now matter how well we chew, tiny bits of the nut, each containing hundreds of thousands of intact cells, will make it down to our colon,[365] where the fat can be released by fiber-eating bacteria to activate GLP-1 secretion. The same happens when we eat an apple or steel-cut oats. Instead of all the sugar and starch getting absorbed earlier, like it would if we drank apple juice or ate a cracker, some of the carbohydrates are released further down our digestive tract to activate our satiety hormones.

The milling of whole grains into flour can break open all the grains' cell walls, but whole-grain bread is still better than bread made with *refined* grains, because whole-grain bread at least has extra fiber that makes it down to our colon. There, our good gut bugs can turn the fiber into short-chain fatty acids that, on their own, can activate GLP-1 secretion.[366] What's more, fiber has a gelling property that can trap other calories in the meal and pull them further down the intestine. Chug a third of a cup of oil on a high-fiber diet, and more than twice as much fat makes it to our colon than if we drank the same amount of oil on a low-fiber diet.[367] In other words, even if we ate a donut on an otherwise high-fiber diet, more of the donut's calories might make it far enough to help dial down our hunger. Dietary fiber can help slow the digestion and absorption of calories so they can make it far enough to activate GLP-1 secretion for satiety.

This "slow digestion strategy" has been proposed as a way to use diet to "mimic the function of bariatric surgery."[368] Because certain surgical procedures can involve literally removing a section of the small intestine, nutrients can skip down to activate the GLP-1 ileal brake response.[369] This may be one of the reasons bariatric surgery can result in long-term weight loss.

So, the modern medical solution to this mismatch between the foods we were built to eat that naturally activate satiety circuits and the processed junk we're now being sold is to (1) physically, surgically change our anatomy to force calories to the end of our gut to activate GLP-1 or (2) inject drugs that mimic GLP-1 so we get GLP-1 activation regardless of what we eat.

It's telling when researchers state that few nutrients make it down to where GLP-1-producing cells are concentrated "under normal situations."[370] By "normal," they mean having donuts for breakfast. But normal-for-our-species is actually eating so many unprocessed plant foods that we reached triple-digit grams of fiber a day. Our Paleolithic intake of fiber was estimated at more than a hundred daily grams,[371] whereas, today, the average daily intake in the United States is only 16 grams.[372]

To restore our natural satiety circuits, we can go under the knife, under the needle, or just eat the way nature intended.

Vinegar to Boost GLP-1

Remember how a tofu burger boosted levels of GLP-1 higher than did a meat burger, even though the two were matched for calories and macronutrients? One thing that may have given the plant-based meal an edge, at least over time, is increased fiber.[373]

When we eat prebiotics like dietary fiber, they can often be fermented by good bacteria in our colon[374] into short-chain fatty acids called acetate, propionate, and butyrate, which then stimulate the release of GLP-1.[375] In contrast, a bacterial breakdown product of tryptophan, which is concentrated in animal protein,[376] has been found to have opposite effects on GLP-1 release.[377]

How do we know fiber-derived short-chain fatty acids boost GLP-1? Higher levels of them in our blood is correlated with higher GLP-1 concentrations, but that doesn't prove cause and effect.[378] For that, researchers needed to stick tubes in people's butts. Rectal infusions of acetate do in fact cause GLP-1 levels to rise in our blood, and the acetate blood concentrations reached after rectal infusion were within an achievable range,[379] in the ballpark of what we'd get eating 15 more grams of fiber a day.[380]

There is a third way to get appetite-suppressing short-chain fatty acids in our bloodstream besides the top-down approach of eating healthy foods and the bottoms-up approach of getting them squirted into our rectum. When vinegar is consumed, its acetic acid is rapidly neutralized into the same acetate our good gut bugs make from fiber.[381] No wonder vinegar has been used to treat obesity for centuries.[382]

To determine if short-chain fatty acids can reduce cravings, researchers scanned people's brains. Propionate, another fiber-derived short-chain fatty acid, was delivered into the colons of study participants while they were shown images of pizzas, cakes, and chocolates. Researchers found that increasing colonic propionate reduced activation in the reward centers of the brain, as well as decreased the subjective appeal of these kinds of foods. They didn't look as appetizing, and that translated into reduced caloric intake at a buffet meal.[383] This effect did not seem to correlate with GLP-1 changes in the blood, though, so it is possible that short-chain fatty acids produced in the colon signal the brain directly through the vagus nerve and reduce appetite that way.[384]

Regardless, does the boost in GLP-1 and the short-term reduction of caloric intake from the direct delivery of propionate to the colon translate into better weight control in overweight adults? Yes, long-term delivery of colonic propionate was found to prevent body weight gain, particularly deep abdominal fat, and may even reduce liver fat in those with fatty liver disease.[385]

Prebiotics to Boost GLP-1

When various prebiotics have been put to the test, they sometimes worked, boosting GLP-1[386] and driving down hunger,[387] but overall, the findings of human interventions with prebiotics have been described as "mixed"[388]— and that's putting it lightly.[389] Certain isolated dietary fibers bump up GLP-1, some drop it down, and others have no effect at all.[390] In some cases, it's possible that macronutrients that would otherwise stimulate GLP-1 might get caught up in viscous, fibrous masses and result in lower GLP-1 levels.[391] Ultimately, results for short-term prebiotic trials are said to be "completely inconclusive for GLP-1."[392]

One explanation may be the dose. In one study, for example, researchers tested refined-grain bread versus whole-grain bread. Although the whole-grain bread improved satiety, it had no effect on GLP-1. The difference in fiber content was only about 5 grams, which may not be enough.[393] In a study in which participants were randomized to get 5 or 10 grams of a fiber supplement called Fibersol, for instance, the 5-gram dose appeared to have no greater effect on GLP-1 than placebo. Only the 10-gram dose worked, which is about two tablespoons. Similarly, there were significant delays in hunger and increased satiety after 10 grams but not 5.[394]

Another issue may be the duration. Studies like these may only last a few hours,[395] but the more fiber-rich foods we eat, the more we foster the growth of more fiber feeders, which can translate into additional GLP-1 secretion over time.[396] As well, eating more fiber-rich foods may even promote the emergence of more GLP-1-secreting cells in our intestinal lining.[397] These may help explain the findings of a randomized controlled trial of different breakfast cereals that lasted a whole year.

People who eat whole grains tend to get less diabetes, but there doesn't seem to be much improvement in blood sugar control after switching to whole wheat for weeks or even months. Might it take longer for our colon to adapt to increased fiber intake? That's what this cereal study found: Study participants were randomized to a year of either All-Bran or Rice Krispies cereal for breakfast. Significant increases in short-chain fatty acid production and GLP-1 secretion were found in the higher fiber group, but it took 9 to 12 months for those benefits to develop.[398]

Finally, it's important to recognize that all dietary fiber is not the same. Fiber is not a single nutrient. There are literally thousands of types of fiber in plant foods, and each one may support different communities of bacteria in our gut.[399] That's the reasoning behind recommendations to take the "50-food challenge" and eat at least 50 different plant foods a week to achieve a diet diverse enough to feed a vast spectrum of gut bacteria.[400]

Those who get more fiber in their diet are significantly less likely to get heart disease and die from it; less likely to get cardiovascular disease in general and less likely to die from it; and less likely to have a stroke, get diabetes, be diagnosed with colorectal cancer, and die from cancer across the board, as well as from all causes put together.[401] All of this associated protection is from getting fiber from food, not supplements. Some types of fiber supplements, like psyllium (Metamucil), can't be fermented by our gut bugs at all,[402] and others don't even exist in nature.

Take Fibersol, for example. Fibersol is a registered trademark of Matsutani Chemical Industry, the company that invented it.[403] Its promotional material includes "innovation success stories" with a photo of a milkshake drizzled with fudge and topped with whipped cream, cookies, marshmallows, *and* a glazed donut, explaining how manufacturers can "increase the fiber content of a finished product."[404] It may be better to stick to foods that were instead invented by Mother Nature.

"Lente" Carbohydrates to Boost GLP-1

Fiber and other prebiotics don't represent the only slow digestion strategy to stimulate GLP-1 secretion.[405] There is a drug called acarbose[406] that acts as a starch blocker by inhibiting the enzymes that would normally digest carbohydrates early in the small intestine. The delay in carbohydrate digestion further down the GI tract leads to an increase in GLP-1 levels that correlates with weight loss in those taking the drug.[407,408]

Instead of taking a drug to slow the digestion of carbs, why not just choose more "lente" carbohydrates, from the Latin *lentus* for "slow." The hope was that comparable effects could be obtained by eating slow-digesting carbohydrates, such as beans, pasta, sprouted grains, and structurally intact grain kernels known as *groats*.[409]

One study on beans showed GLP-1-boosting effects—bread made with coarsely ground chickpea flour raised GLP-1 higher than bread without[410]—but another did not. Asking people to eat five cups of beans a week spontaneously led to a variety of health benefits, but there was no change in GLP-1 levels.[411] What about *cocoa* beans? Unfortunately, dark chocolate didn't have an effect on GLP-1 either.[412]

I found only one study on pasta, which also failed to raise GLP-1,[413] but the one sprouted grain study I found did show a higher GLP-1 response to sprouted grain bread compared to four other bread types, which didn't differ significantly from each other.[414] You may be surprised that 11- or 12-grain bread was no different than white bread, but that's the general finding when comparing products made with whole-grain flour to refined-grain flour.[415] There are few short-term differences in how our body reacts to whole-wheat bread compared to white bread, for example. Unlike eating sprouted grain bread, which can be made without powdering the grains, we can't eat bread made out of flour and expect some kind of *doughzempic* effect. When grains—whether whole wheat or white—are milled into flour, their cell walls are ruptured and the starch spills out, never making it down to our colon to activate GLP-1 production.

This is one of the reasons that Walter C. Willett, the former chair of Harvard's nutrition department, has argued that the term *whole grain* should probably be reserved for only groats, intact grain kernels,[416] the wholiest of grains. In my book *How Not to Diet*, I talked about my BROL bowl, a prebiotic mix that includes barley groats, rye groats, and oat groats. What effect might they have on GLP-1?

Groatzempic: Intact Grains to Boost GLP-1

If we eat bread containing some whole, intact barley groats, there's no immediate difference in GLP-1 levels in the subsequent three hours—but that wouldn't be enough time for the groats to make it down to our colon. However, after our good bacteria have had a chance to break open the groats' cell walls, we get a GLP-1 bump more than 12 hours later, at breakfast the next day.[417]

Researchers found that this also translates into a suppressed appetite. Having barley kernels at an evening meal not only boosted GLP-1 blood levels by 43 percent at breakfast, but feelings of hunger were also decreased during that entire next day. The study participants ate less breakfast, as well as about 100 fewer calories of an all-you-can-eat lunch—simply because they had eaten some barley groats 14 hours before.[418]

And the more, the merrier. Three consecutive days of consuming barley groats led to a 56 percent increase in the level of GLP-1 in the blood by day four.[419]

This effect isn't restricted to barley groats. When rye groats were eaten at dinner, GLP-1 levels were up and appetite down more than ten hours later. Researchers similarly found that participants had an increased subjective feeling of satiety during the entire next day. There was a correlation between short-chain fatty acid blood levels and the GLP-1 response, suggesting that, indeed, we have our good gut bugs to thank for the beneficial effects.[420]

Thylakoids to Boost GLP-1

Thylakoids are the chlorophyll-rich membranes inside leaves where photosynthesis takes place. They act as fat blockers, delaying our digestion of fats and promoting the release of satiety hormones like GLP-1.[421]

When we eat thylakoids, when we bite into a leaf of spinach, for instance, the thylakoid membranes are able to resist our digestive enzymes. They can last for hours in our gut before finally getting broken down,[422] and it is in those hours that they work their magic. Thylakoids glom onto and surround tiny droplets of fat in our digestive tract,[423] and, in this way, powerfully slow our digestion of fats, which means more GLP-1 activation in the end. Compared to drugs, thylakoids are described as "an easier and more physiological way to enhance GLP-1 levels to achieve satiety and energy balance."[424] Are they saying that eating some kale could actually cut cravings? Yes.

Cutting Cravings with Thylakoids

Researchers disguised spinach extracts in jam[425] and juice[426] to sneak thylakoids undetected into meals. Study participants who unwittingly ate the equivalent of about half a cup of cooked spinach felt significantly less hungry and more satiated over the next few hours. Having the equivalent of a shot of wheatgrass juice or what might be in a green juice or green smoothie not only left people more satiated, but their cravings for sweet, salty, and fatty snacks, such as potato chips, chocolate, and cinnamon buns, dropped by about a third. When they were given candy anyway, those who had unknowingly consumed the spinach reported liking the sweets significantly less.[427] The satiating power of greens has been attributed to their low calorie density and high fiber and water contents,[428] but the thylakoids may be their secret weapon, presumably because of an increase in GLP-1 release after consuming them.

In a systematic review of randomized clinical trials on the effects of thylakoid intake on appetite and weight loss, hunger-suppressing effects of thylakoids were reported across the board.[429] And weight loss? Would the GLP-induced reduction of cravings and hunger from greens translate into losing pounds?

Losing Weight with Thylakoids

A single morning dose of thylakoids can decrease hunger and cravings for snacks and sweets throughout the day. After one dose of greens, researchers found significantly less wanting of salty snacks over the next nine hours, compared to placebo, and significantly less wanting of sweet snacks, sweets and fats, and snacks in general.[430] Thylakoids are described as a "powerful strategy to suppress the urge for palatable food."[431] Despite lower reported hunger and greater reported satiety, food intake throughout the day was not significantly affected.[432] Instead of having a single dose of greens, what about getting the same dose every day for months?

This study title says it all: "Body Weight Loss, Reduced Urge for Palatable Food and Increased Release of GLP-1 Through Daily Supplementation with Green-Plant Membranes for Three Months in Overweight Women."[433] The average amount of weight loss was only about three pounds, but the study participants also experienced a significant drop in cholesterol of 20 points. And the drop in cholesterol preceded significant weight loss, so the cholesterol benefit wasn't just due to losing weight. A 20-point drop in cholesterol is meaningful, comparable to what is achieved with a class of cholesterol-lowering drugs known as *bile acid sequestrants*.

GLP-1 was also boosted by about 40 percent, and there were significantly lower cravings for sweets *11 hours* after spinach intake. And remember: The spinach powder was hidden, so people didn't know if they were getting greens or placebo, yet 11 hours after a single dose, cravings for chocolate were found to be significantly lower in the greens group. That's the power of GLP-1.[434]

One of the authors of the study had a conflict of interest, though: affiliations with companies commercializing thylakoid products. You can smell the bias by how the results were spun. The spinach extract was described as "markedly" reducing body weight, but three pounds in three months isn't that remarkable. The authors boasted the 6 percent weight loss was comparable to the older GLP-1 drug available at the time, suggesting that thylakoids "may be as efficient for obesity treatment as pharmacological agents." But, of course, newer GLP-1 drugs can decrease body weight by more than 6 percent, and that 6 percent loss in this study was from baseline, not compared to placebo. Those on the placebo lost about 4 percent of their body weight, so the weight loss attributable to the spinach was closer to 2 percent. What's more, a shorter eight-week study found no significant difference at all.[435]

So, when one of the companies took its thylakoid supplement to the European equivalent of the FDA to try to make a weight-loss health claim, the Panel rebuffed its petition, given how underwhelming the weight loss was.[436] Since then, a third study was published, a randomized, double-blind, placebo-controlled trial with that same dose-equivalent to half a cup of cooked greens. Those researchers found a significant decrease in body weight, waist circumference, fat mass, BMI, and waist-to-height ratio, compared to the placebo—and by a decent amount. Individuals in the spinach group lost 8 more pounds than those in the placebo group over three months—15 pounds lost versus 7. And that appeared to be 8 pounds of straight fat, along with four more centimeters off the waist, compared to placebo.[437]

Interestingly, supplementing a breakfast that was only 11 percent fat with thylakoids was also shown to result in reduced hunger and cravings.[438] This suggests the appetite-suppressing effect of thylakoids may have other mechanisms beyond simply slowing the digestion of fat,[439] such as improving our gut microbiota.[440]

In summary, a systematic review of the potential role of thylakoids in the management of obesity concluded that "eating green" can suppress hunger, reduce food intake, and result in weight loss.[441] Consuming the thylakoids in dark green leafy vegetables is said to "offer a means to strengthen the resolve to refrain from eating especially in an environment where there is superfluous access to foods processed to deliver qualities that some may find irresistible."[442]

Choosing the Best Greens to Boost GLP-1

The best way to get thylakoids is not from the supplement aisle, but the produce department. Since thylakoids are where chlorophyll is found, we can see with our own eyes which veggies have the most. The darker our dark leafy greens, the better.[443]

What happens when we cook greens? Blanched for 15 seconds or so in steaming or boiling water, they turn an even brighter green, but if cooked too long, they eventually become a drab olive brown. When greens are overcooked, their thylakoids physically degrade, along with their ability to slow fat absorption.

But, within that first minute of cooking, when the green gets even more vibrant, there is a slight boost in fat-blocking ability.[444] So we can gauge thylakoid activity in both the grocery store and in our kitchen just by sight.

continued

We have been eating leaves for millions of years,[445] but, today, the greenest thing about some of our diets may be a St. Patrick's Day pint. Americans average less than 2 grams of spinach a day. That isn't even half a teaspoon.[446] But our bodies were designed to have thylakoids passing through our system on a daily basis, so that delay in fat absorption we get from them can be thought of as our default, normal state.[447] It's only when we eat diets deficient in greens that we suffer accelerated digestion of fat that undercuts our natural satiety mechanisms. In the journal of the Society of Chemical Industry, a group of food technologists argued that, given the fat-blocking benefits of thylakoids, they "could be incorporated in functional foods as a new promising appetite-reducing ingredient."[448] Yes, or we can just get them from the produce aisle.

TREATING THE PRIMARY CAUSE
OF OBESITY

"Game Changers: Do New Medications Make Lifestyle-Based Treatment of Obesity Obsolete?" was the question asked by the title of an article in the medical journal *Obesity*,[449] written by researchers personally paid by the two main GLP-1 drug manufacturers, which now have a combined net worth in excess of a trillion dollars.[450] An episode of *60 Minutes*, "America's #1 television news program," certainly seemed to think so.[451] Only later did we learn that Novo Nordisk, the makers of Ozempic, evidently paid *60 Minutes* to air the 13-minute promotional segment and pass it off as a news story. The president of the European Association for the Study of Obesity was also pretty bullish in an editorial in *The Guardian*, conveniently failing to disclose that his organization had received millions of dollars from the drug maker.[452]

Novo Nordisk also reportedly made a funding commitment of a million dollars to the World Obesity Federation, which then published a "consensus statement" arguing that obesity itself should be defined as a disease.[453] Designating obesity a disease may benefit Big Pharma more than it does big people. A concern is that labelling obesity as a disease "risks reducing autonomy, disempowering and robbing people of the intrinsic motivation that is such an important enabler of change. It encourages fatalism, promoting the fallacy that genetics are destiny."[454]

Of course, it can't all be our genes. The obesity epidemic only started a few decades ago,[455] and our genes didn't somehow magically change in the late 1970s.[456] Others blame a lack of willpower,[457] but that doesn't make sense either. We all—suddenly and coincidentally—lost all our collective self-control?[458]

Obesity is not a disease caused by a GLP-1 hormone deficiency. It's the food.

A Toxic Food Environment

The rise in the number of excess calories provided by the food supply is more than sufficient to explain the obesity epidemic.[459] Obesity is not some moral failing. The battle of the bulge is a battle against biology. We're drowning in a sea of excess calories while being bombarded with ads for fast food and candy.[460] Becoming overweight is a normal, natural response to the abnormal, unnatural ubiquity of sugary, fatty foods that are concentrated with calories.[461]

The prime cause for the obesity epidemic is neither gluttony nor sloth. Being overweight may simply be "a normal response, by normal people, to an abnormal situation."[462] And with so many of us overweight— nearly three-quarters of Americans, for example—it's *literally* normal.[463]

If obesity is to be understood as "normal physiology within a pathological environment,"[464] it can be argued that drugs like Ozempic really aren't tackling its root cause.[465] In that case, these drugs will likely have only a modest effect on the obesity epidemic—and could potentially make it even worse. The pharmaceutical industry and its lobbyists continue to try to shift society's focus to drugs, rather than broader public health strategies. The real solution involves fixing the broken food system, but, as an editorial in the leading medical ethics journal asked, "why would Big Food change its ways if obesity can be treated with drugs?"[466]

England's health secretary was keen to use GLP-1 drugs as "a way of preventing illness without resorting to 'nanny state' measures,"[467] but most public health advocates are mainly talking about measures such as restricting the thousands of commercials children see every year for candy, liquid candy (soft drinks), breakfast candy (sugary cereals), and fast food.[468]

Commercial Influence

A quarter century ago, the term "Social Determinants of Health" was coined,[469] defined as the *non*medical factors influencing health,[470] such as poverty, that are too often ignored by the medical establishment. They help explain why the richest 1 percent, for example, live about 10 to 15 years longer than the poorest 1 percent.[471]

More recently, based on experiences with the alcohol and tobacco industries, the concept of "commercial determinants of health" was introduced, defined as "factors that influence health which stem from the profit motive,"[472] also known as "corporate determinants of health." The effects of the food and beverage sector is framed as a prime example, spending billions on marketing products that are "deliberately designed to lead to addictive consumption," which contribute to a pandemic of chronic disease.[473] As one public health researcher concluded in an *Addiction* journal commentary, "The greatest challenge to improving health may lie in the tension between wealth- and health-creation."[474]

Baked into the Formula

The *Drug and Therapeutics Bulletin* is one of the most respected sources of independent information about medications.[475] It concluded that more data on semaglutide's long-term safety and efficacy are needed before it can be recommended for routine use in treating obesity, reminding readers that, historically, nearly all the drugs approved for weight loss have later been pulled from the market because of safety concerns.[476]

From a commissioned feature on semaglutide in the *British Medical Journal*: "Historically, the medical profession has offered a sorry collection of non-evidenced, harmful, or downright dangerous interventions to often desperate people. Caution about long-term side effects is therefore warranted...."[477] Consider the past withdrawals of anti-obesity drugs from the market, pulled because of safety concerns only discovered years after they had been approved. It took an average of a decade before dangers came to light. In one case, a weight-loss drug's long-term adverse effects weren't discovered until 38 years after it hit the market. What's more, even after that first report of danger, it takes an average of another decade for that drug to actually get banned, or even as long as another two decades even though people lost their lives in about a quarter of the cases.[478] As one critic said about how long it takes regulators to act, "It would probably take the system 2 years to ban cyanide."[479]

It's all baked into the formula. In the journal *PharmacoEconomics*, papers like "The Expected Net Present Value of Developing Weight Management Drugs in the Context of Drug Safety Litigation" estimate that new weight-loss drugs may injure or kill so many that "expected litigation cost" could exceed $80 million. But, if successful, the drug could bring in more than $100 million.[480] Pharma can do the math.

In December 2023, for example, a French drug maker was fined nearly half a billion dollars for fraud and relentlessly promoting its appetite-suppressing weight-loss drug while covering up known harms,[481] causing hundreds or even thousands of people to die from heart valve problems.[482] It made up to €20 million a year for the 33 years its drug was on the market,[483] though. It was fined €430 million but may have made up to €660 million.[484] Did it learn its lesson? (These days, GLP-1 drug makers are worth more than a *trillion* dollars. Do you think they'd ever try to cover anything up?[485])

Obesity so dramatically decreases one's lifespan[486] that, even if these drugs ended up shaving literally years off people's lives, wouldn't they still be worth it? That assumes these drugs cure obesity, though. If you remember, in all the major research trials, individuals taking the drug started out obese and ended up obese, no matter how long they were on them because the medications effectively stop working as body weight plateaus. They are then left paying for a lifetime of prescriptions just to avoid re-gaining the lost weight, while continuing to face any and all short- and long-term side effects.

Tackling the Root Cause of Obesity

Using GLP-1 drugs as a temporary weight-loss fix has been likened to "sprinkling teaspoons of water onto an increasing blaze."[487] The war against obesity cannot be won without measures to prevent obesity in the first place.[488] That means tackling the food environment, which, today, is largely based on high-calorie, fatty, salty, sugary junk, rather than relying on medication as a "damage limitation exercise."[489]

But isn't limiting damage a good thing? These drugs may not make much of a dent on a population scale, but what about on an individual basis?

Ideally, we would eat healthfully enough to prevent and treat heart disease, high blood pressure, and diabetes, too, but until that happens, drugs for those conditions can literally be lifesaving. Obesity so diminishes one's lifespan—reducing life expectancy as much as a decade—that these GLP-1 drugs, just like bariatric surgery, should be considered as a last resort for those unwilling or unable to treat the cause of their obesity.[490]

The problem is we eat too much crap, so anything that gets us to eat less crap can be beneficial, including surgically rearranging our digestive organs. Studies show that people with diabetes on Ozempic eat less high-fat and sweet foods,[491] like pastries and donuts, and people without diabetes on Ozempic eat less high-fat and savory foods, like sausages and cheese.[492] But we don't need to go under the knife or take expensive drugs to decrap our diet.

What about cravings? Pharmaceutical industry–funded representatives argue that GLP-1 drugs are necessary because the obesogenic—obesity-generating—toxic food environment "will overwhelm even substantial efforts...to enact individual behavior changes."[493] After ramping up for three months to high-dose Ozempic for weight loss, people are able to cut nearly a thousand calories out of their daily diet.[494] How could you possibly do that without drugs, unless you did some sort of liquid diet, meal replacement shakes or something?

You could eat a diet centered around the healthiest foods on the planet.

Plants, Not Pills

When study participants were placed on a diet packed with fruits, vegetables, whole grains, and beans and allowed to eat as much as they wanted, they end up eating about 50 percent fewer calories than they might have otherwise.[495] They were just as full, on half the calories. How is it possible that people could be satisfied after cutting more than a thousand calories out of their diet each day? By emphasizing "large quantities of high-bulk low-energy-density foods (primarily vegetables, fruits, high-fiber grains, and cereals) and moderation in high energy-density foods (meats, cheeses, sugars, and fats)."[496] It's no wonder whole food, plant-based nutrition has been proven to be one of the most powerful dietary weight-loss interventions.[497] And, as I've described, adding groats, greens, and certain spices may provide an extra GLP-1 boost.

So, good nutrition may present a safer and cheaper approach to weight loss for most patients. Not only can the ingestion of a plant-based meal more than double GLP-1 secretion, compared to a meat meal, but plant-based diets can also cause weight loss by boosting our resting metabolic rate and incorporating "calorie-trapping" high-fiber foods that flush calories away. The largest study of people eating strictly plant-based found they are about 35 pounds lighter on average. And in contrast to the exorbitant costs of these new weight-loss drugs, eating more healthfully can actually save money.[498] More plant-based diets have been found to be up to 25 to 29 percent less expensive.[499]

CONCLUSION

When we eat a donut, its fat, sugar, and starch get absorbed quickly, high up, before reaching the part of our digestive tract where we produce most of the hormone that suppresses our appetite, GLP-1. Since the cells that produce GLP-1 in response to calorie exposure are concentrated at the end of our digestive tract, while the majority of the calories we consume are absorbed early on,[500] most calories never make it down far enough. That's why our appetites aren't suppressed very much these days. From a GLP-1 standpoint, when we have that donut, it's like we never ate much of anything. No wonder we reach for donut number two.

Our medical system has some solutions, though. How can we eat a donut and still get GLP-1 activation? Surgery! Why not undergo bariatric surgery and cut out part of the small intestine so some donut calories make it to the end of the GI tract after all? What if we want to eat a donut, still get GLP-1 activation, and keep our anatomy intact? Drugs! Acarbose, the starch blocker that slows the digestion of carbohydrates, or the drug orlistat, the fat blocker that slows the digestion of fats, could raise GLP-1 on a donut diet. Or we can just inject drugs like Ozempic that mimic GLP-1 and get GLP-1 activation no matter what we eat.

What if we want GLP-1 activation without drugs or surgery? Well, we could try not eating donuts.

Our prehistoric ancestors are believed to have consumed as much as 100 daily grams of fiber, which is more than six times what most of us are getting these days. We evolved eating massive amounts of whole plant foods—the only places fiber is found in abundance.[501] That enabled our natural satiety mechanisms to keep us from overeating.

By eating the way nature intended, we can release GLP-1 the way nature intended. That helps explains why in the medical literature, compared to any other way of eating that didn't involve portion control, a whole food, plant-based diet has been shown to lead to greater average weight loss than any other diet.[502]

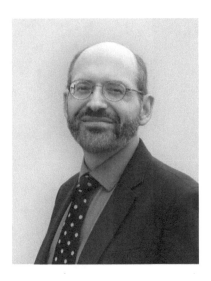

A founding member and fellow of the American College of Lifestyle Medicine, **DR. MICHAEL GREGER** is a physician, *New York Times* bestselling author, internationally recognized speaker on nutrition, and founder of the acclaimed nonprofit public health organization, NutritionFacts.org. He is a graduate of the Cornell University College of Agriculture and Life Sciences and Tufts University School of Medicine.

All of the proceeds he receives from his books and speaking engagements are donated to charity.

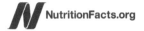

NOTES

1. Klitzman R, Greenberg H. Anti-obesity medications: ethical, policy, and public health concerns. *Hastings Cent Rep*. 2024;54(3):6–10.

2. Thorp HH. More questions than answers. *Science*. 2023;382(6676):1213.

3. Klitzman R, Greenberg H. Anti-obesity medications: ethical, policy, and public health concerns. *Hastings Cent Rep*. 2024;54(3):6–10.

4. Lewis KH, Moore JB, Ard JD. Game changers: do new medications make lifestyle-based treatment of obesity obsolete? *Obesity (Silver Spring)*. 2024;32(2):237–9.

5. Spector R. A revolution in the treatment of obesity. *Am J Med*. Published online May 22, 2024:S0002-9343(24)00334-6.

6. Holst JJ. Glucagon-like peptide-1: are its roles as endogenous hormone and therapeutic wizard congruent? *J Intern Med*. 2022;291(5):557–73.

7. Gong B, Yao Z, Zhou C, Wang W, Sun L, Han J. Glucagon-like peptide-1 analogs: miracle drugs are blooming? *Eur J Med Chem*. 2024;269:116342.

8. Dowsett GKC, Yeo GSH. Are GLP-1R agonists the long-sought-after panacea for obesity? *Trends Mol Med*. 2023;29(10):777–9.

9. Müller TD, Finan B, Bloom SR, et al. Glucagon-like peptide 1 (GLP-1). *Mol Metab*. 2019;30:72–130.

10. Onakpoya IJ, Heneghan CJ, Aronson JK. Post-marketing withdrawal of anti-obesity medicinal products because of adverse drug reactions: a systematic review. *BMC Med*. 2016;14(1):191.

11. Couzin-Frankel J. Obesity meets its match. *Science*. 2023;382(6676):1226–7.

12. For more on this, see *Are Weight-Loss Pills Safe?* at see.nf/pills.

13. Wharton S, Serodio KJ. Next generation of weight management medications: implications for diabetes and CVD risk. *Curr Cardiol Rep*. 2015;17(5):35.

14. McGee M, Whitehead N, Martin J, Collins N. Drug-associated pulmonary arterial hypertension. *Clin Toxicol (Phila)*. 2018;56(9):801–9.

15. Kassirer JP, Angell M. Losing weight—an ill-fated New Year's resolution. *N Engl J Med*. 1998;338(1):52–4.

16. Connolly HM, Crary JL, McGoon MD, et al. Valvular heart disease associated with fenfluramine-phentermine. *N Engl J Med*. 1997;337(9):581–8.

17. James WP, Caterson ID, Coutinho W, et al. Effect of sibutramine on cardiovascular outcomes in overweight and obese subjects. *N Engl J Med*. 2010;363(10):905–17.

18. Christensen R, Kristensen PK, Bartels EM, Bliddal H, Astrup A. Efficacy and safety of the weight-loss drug rimonabant: a meta-analysis of randomised trials. *Lancet*. 2007;370(9600):1706–13.

19. U.S. Food and Drug Administration. FDA requests the withdrawal of the weight-loss drug Belviq, Belviq XR (lorcaserin) from the market. FDA.org. Feb 13, 2020. Accessed Sept 10, 2024. https://www.fda.gov/drugs/drug-safety-and-availability/fda-requests-withdrawal-weight-loss-drug-belviq-belviq-xr-lorcaserin-market

20. Tak YJ, Lee SY. Long-term efficacy and safety of anti-obesity treatment: where do we stand? *Curr Obes Rep*. 2021;10(1):14–30.

21. Kumar R, Ryan D. Lorcaserin departs, leaving more questions than answers. *Obesity (Silver Spring)*. 2020;28(7):1167.

22. Moyad MA. Embracing the pros and cons of the new weight loss medications (semaglutide, tirzepatide, etc.). *Curr Urol Rep*. 2023;24(11):515–25.

23. Diet, drugs, devices, and surgery for weight management. *Med Lett Drugs Ther*. 2018;60(1548):91–8.

24. Igel LI, Kumar RB, Saunders KH, Aronne LJ. Practical use of pharmacotherapy for obesity. *Gastroenterology*. 2017;152(7):1765–79.

25. Igel LI, Kumar RB, Saunders KH, Aronne LJ. Practical use of pharmacotherapy for obesity. *Gastroenterology*. 2017;152(7):1765–79.

26. Shepherd RW. No evidence for benefit of medication for obesity. *Can Fam Physician*. 2017;63(4):276.

27. Shi Q, Wang Y, Hao Q, et al. Pharmacotherapy for adults with overweight and obesity: a systematic review and network meta-analysis of randomised controlled trials. *Lancet*. 2024;403(10434):e21–31.

28. Moyad MA. Embracing the pros and cons of the new weight loss medications (semaglutide, tirzepatide, etc.). *Curr Urol Rep*. 2023;24(11):515–25.

29. Shi Q, Wang Y, Hao Q, et al. Pharmacotherapy for adults with overweight and obesity: a systematic review and network meta-analysis of randomised controlled trials. *Lancet*. 2024;403(10434):e21–31.

30. Schmitz SH, Aronne LJ. The effective use of anti-obesity medications. *Gastroenterol Clin North Am*. 2023;52(4):661–80.

31. Qi QYD, Cox A, McNeil S, Sumithran P. Obesity medications: a narrative review of current and emerging agents. *Osteoarthr Cartil Open*. 2024;6(2):100472.

32. Moyad MA. Embracing the pros and cons of the new weight loss medications (semaglutide, tirzepatide, etc.). *Curr Urol Rep*. 2023;24(11):515–25.

33. Hong SH, Choi KM. Gut hormones and appetite regulation. *Curr Opin Endocrinol Diabetes Obes*. 2024;31(3):115–21.

34. Angelini G, Russo S, Mingrone G. Incretin hormones, obesity and gut microbiota. *Peptides*. 2024;178:171216.

35. Holst JJ. Glucagon-like peptide-1: are its roles as endogenous hormone and therapeutic wizard congruent? *J Intern Med*. 2022;291(5):557–73.

36. Drucker DJ, Holst JJ. The expanding incretin universe: from basic biology to clinical translation. *Diabetologia*. 2023;66(10):1765–79.

37. Prillaman M. Four key questions on the new wave of anti-obesity drugs. *Nature*. 2023;620(7972):28–30.

38. Gong B, Yao Z, Zhou C, Wang W, Sun L, Han J. Glucagon-like peptide-1 analogs: miracle drugs are blooming? *Eur J Med Chem*. 2024;269:116342.

39. Holst JJ. Glucagon-like peptide-1: are its roles as endogenous hormone and therapeutic wizard congruent? *J Intern Med*. 2022;291(5):557–73.

40. Krook A, Mulder H. Incretins: turning the venom into the antidote. *Diabetologia*. 2023;66(10):1762–4.

41. Brandfon S, Eylon A, Khanna D, Parmar MS. Advances in anti-obesity pharmacotherapy: current treatments, emerging therapies, and challenges. *Cureus*. 2023;15(10):e46623.

42. Suran M. As Ozempic's popularity soars, here's what to know about semaglutide and weight loss. *JAMA*. 2023;329(19):1627–9.

43. Prillaman M. Four key questions on the new wave of anti-obesity drugs. *Nature*. 2023;620(7972):28–30.

44. Kokkorakis M, Katsarou A, Katsiki N, Mantzoros CS. Milestones in the journey towards addressing obesity; past trials and triumphs, recent breakthroughs, and an exciting future in the era of emerging effective medical therapies and integration of effective medical therapies with metabolic surgery. *Metabolism*. 2023;148:155689.

45. Moyad MA. Embracing the pros and cons of the new weight loss medications (semaglutide, tirzepatide, etc.). *Curr Urol Rep*. 2023;24(11):515–25.

46. Mullard A. Mediator scandal rocks French medical community. *Lancet*. 2011;377(9769):890–2.

47. Frachon I, Benkimoun P. Tough ruling for Servier in the Mediator trial. *Lancet*. 2024;403(10433):1235–6.

48. Suran M. As Ozempic's popularity soars, here's what to know about semaglutide and weight loss. *JAMA*. 2023;329(19):1627–9.

49. Kokkorakis M, Katsarou A, Katsiki N, Mantzoros CS. Milestones in the journey towards addressing obesity; past trials and triumphs, recent breakthroughs, and an exciting future in the era of emerging effective medical therapies and integration of effective medical therapies with metabolic surgery. *Metabolism*. 2023;148:155689.

50. Graham S, Fraser IS. The progestogen-only mini-pill. *Contraception*. 1982;26(4):373–88.

51. Suran M. As Ozempic's popularity soars, here's what to know about semaglutide and weight loss. *JAMA*. 2023;329(19):1627–9.

52. Jewell ML. Commentary on: aesthetic surgery journal articles on injectable weight loss medications and their role in plastic surgery. *Aesthet Surg J*. 2023;44(1):80–3.

53. Suran M. As Ozempic's popularity soars, here's what to know about semaglutide and weight loss. *JAMA*. 2023;329(19):1627–9.

54. Moyad MA. Embracing the pros and cons of the new weight loss medications (semaglutide, tirzepatide, etc.). *Curr Urol Rep*. 2023;24(11):515–25.

55. Mozaffarian D. GLP-1 agonists for obesity—a new recipe for success? *JAMA*. 2024;331(12):1007–8.

56. Haddock CK, Poston WSC, Dill PL, Foreyt JP, Ericsson M. Pharmacotherapy for obesity: a quantitative analysis of four decades of published randomized clinical trials. *Int J Obes Relat Metab Disord*. 2002;26(2):262–73.

57. Ansari HUH, Qazi SU, Sajid F, et al. Efficacy and safety of glucagon-like peptide-1 receptor agonists on body weight and cardiometabolic parameters in individuals with obesity and without diabetes: a systematic review and meta-analysis. *Endocr Pract*. 2024;30(2):160–71.

58. Qin W, Yang J, Deng C, Ruan Q, Duan K. Efficacy and safety of semaglutide 2.4 mg for weight loss in overweight or obese adults without diabetes: an updated systematic review and meta-analysis including the 2-year STEP 5 trial. *Diabetes Obes Metab*. 2024;26(3):911–23.

59. Arvanitakis M. No more needles: oral semaglutide for weight loss. *Gastroenterology*. 2024;166(6):1190–1.

60. Seijas-Amigo J, Salgado-Barreira Á, Castelo-Dominguez R, et al. Differences in weight loss and safety between the glucagon-like peptide-1 receptor agonists: a non-randomized multicenter study from the titration phase. *Prim Care Diabetes*. 2023;17(4):366–72.

61. Liu L, Shi H, Xie M, Sun Y, Nahata MC. Efficacy and safety of tirzepatide versus placebo in overweight or obese adults without diabetes: a systematic review and meta-analysis of randomized controlled trials. *Int J Clin Pharm*. Published online July 22, 2024.

62. Singh A, Nissen SE. Contemporary management of obesity: a comparison of bariatric metabolic surgery and novel incretin mimetic drugs. *Diabetes Technol Ther*. Published online May 16, 2024.

63. Kokkorakis M, Katsarou A, Katsiki N, Mantzoros CS. Milestones in the journey towards addressing obesity; past trials and triumphs, recent breakthroughs, and an exciting future in the era of emerging effective medical therapies and integration of effective medical therapies with metabolic surgery. *Metabolism*. 2023;148:155689.

64. Prillaman M. Obesity drugs aren't always forever. What happens when you quit? *Nature*. 2024;628(8008):488–90.

65. Tzoulis P, Baldeweg SE. Semaglutide for weight loss: unanswered questions. *Front Endocrinol (Lausanne)*. 2024;15:1382814.

66. Ryan DH, Lingvay I, Deanfield J, et al. Long-term weight loss effects of semaglutide in obesity without diabetes in the SELECT trial. *Nat Med*. 2024;30(7):2049–57.

67. Singh A, Nissen SE. Contemporary management of obesity: a comparison of bariatric metabolic surgery and novel incretin mimetic drugs. *Diabetes Technol Ther*. Published online May 16, 2024.

68. Ryan DH, Lingvay I, Deanfield J, et al. Long-term weight loss effects of semaglutide in obesity without diabetes in the SELECT trial. *Nat Med*. 2024;30(7):2049–57.

69. Wilding JPH, Batterham RL, Calanna S, et al. Once-weekly semaglutide in adults with overweight or obesity. *N Engl J Med*. 2021;384(11):989–1002.

70. Davies M, Færch L, Jeppesen OK, et al. Semaglutide 2·4 mg once a week in adults with overweight or obesity, and type 2 diabetes (STEP 2): a randomised, double-blind, double-dummy, placebo-controlled, phase 3 trial. *Lancet*. 2021;397(10278):971–84.

71. Wadden TA, Bailey TS, Billings LK, et al. Effect of subcutaneous semaglutide vs placebo as an adjunct to intensive behavioral therapy on body weight in adults with overweight or obesity: the STEP 3 randomized clinical trial. *JAMA*. 2021;325(14):1403–13.

72. Wilding JPH, Batterham RL, Calanna S, et al. Once-weekly semaglutide in adults with overweight or obesity. *N Engl J Med*. 2021;384(11):989–1002.

73. Davies M, Færch L, Jeppesen OK, et al. Semaglutide 2·4 mg once a week in adults with overweight or obesity, and type 2 diabetes (STEP 2): a randomised, double-blind, double-dummy, placebo-controlled, phase 3 trial. *Lancet*. 2021;397(10278):971–84.

74. Wadden TA, Bailey TS, Billings LK, et al. Effect of subcutaneous semaglutide vs placebo as an adjunct to intensive behavioral therapy on body weight in adults with overweight or obesity: the STEP 3 randomized clinical trial. *JAMA*. 2021;325(14):1403–13.

75. Klitzman R, Greenberg H. Anti-obesity medications: ethical, policy, and public health concerns. *Hastings Cent Rep*. 2024;54(3):6–10.

76. Ruder K. As semaglutide's popularity soars, rare but serious adverse effects are emerging. *JAMA*. 2023;330(22):2140–2.

77. Hall KD. Physiology of the weight-loss plateau in response to diet restriction, GLP-1 receptor agonism, and bariatric surgery. *Obesity (Silver Spring)*. 2024;32(6):1163–8.

78. Hall KD. Physiology of the weight-loss plateau in response to diet restriction, GLP-1 receptor agonism, and bariatric surgery. *Obesity (Silver Spring)*. 2024;32(6):1163–8.

79. Rubino D, Abrahamsson N, Davies M, et al. Effect of continued weekly subcutaneous semaglutide vs placebo on weight loss maintenance in adults with overweight or obesity: the STEP 4 randomized clinical trial. *JAMA*. 2021;325(14):1414–25.

80. Aronne LJ, Sattar N, Horn DB, et al. Continued treatment with tirzepatide for maintenance of weight reduction in adults with obesity: the SURMOUNT-4 randomized clinical trial. *JAMA*. 2024;331(1):38–48.

81. Rubino D, Abrahamsson N, Davies M, et al. Effect of continued weekly subcutaneous semaglutide vs placebo on weight loss maintenance in adults with overweight or obesity: the STEP 4 randomized clinical trial. *JAMA*. 2021;325(14):1414–25.

82. Wilding JPH, Batterham RL, Davies M, et al. Weight regain and cardiometabolic effects after withdrawal of semaglutide: the STEP 1 trial extension. *Diabetes Obes Metab*. 2022;24(8):1553–64.

83. Suran M. As Ozempic's popularity soars, here's what to know about semaglutide and weight loss. *JAMA*. 2023;329(19):1627–9.

84. Klitzman R, Greenberg H. Anti-obesity medications: ethical, policy, and public health concerns. *Hastings Cent Rep*. 2024;54(3):6–10.

85. Suran M. As Ozempic's popularity soars, here's what to know about semaglutide and weight loss. *JAMA*. 2023;329(19):1627–9.

86. Mozaffarian D. GLP-1 agonists for obesity—a new recipe for success? *JAMA*. 2024;331(12):1007–8.

87. Novo Nordisk. Adult dose escalation schedule | Wegovy® (semaglutide) injection 2.4 mg. novoMEDLINK.com. Accessed September 12, 2024. https://www.novomedlink.com/obesity/products/treatments/wegovy/dosing-administration/wegovy-dosing.html

88. Lilly. Your weekly Zepbound routine. Zepbound.Lilly.com. Accessed September 12, 2024. https://zepbound.lilly.com/how-to-use

89. Real-world trends in GLP-1 treatment persistence and prescribing for weight management. *Blue Health Intelligence*. May 2024. Accessed September 23, 2024. https://www.bcbs.com/media/pdf/BHI_Issue_Brief_GLP1_Trends.pdf

90. Prillaman M. Obesity drugs aren't always forever. What happens when you quit? *Nature*. 2024;628(8008):488–90.

91. Klitzman R, Greenberg H. Anti-obesity medications: ethical, policy, and public health concerns. *Hastings Cent Rep*. 2024;54(3):6–10.

92. Lupianez-Merly C, Dilmaghani S, Vosoughi K, Camilleri M. Review article: Pharmacologic management of obesity—updates on approved medications, indications and risks. *Aliment Pharmacol Ther*. 2024;59(4):475–91.

93. Mozaffarian D. GLP-1 agonists for obesity—a new recipe for success? *JAMA*. 2024;331(12):1007–8.

94. Mozaffarian D. GLP-1 agonists for obesity—a new recipe for success? *JAMA*. 2024;331(12):1007–8.

95. Smith G, Muller M. Novo says Ozempic 'very likely' target for next US price cut. *Bloomberg.*September 17, 2024. Accessed September 23, 2024. https://www.bloomberg.com/news/articles/2024-09-17/ozempic-very-likely-to-face-drug-price-negotiations-novo-says

96. Mozaffarian D. GLP-1 agonists for obesity—a new recipe for success? *JAMA.* 2024;331(12):1007–8.

97. Real-world trends in GLP-1 treatment persistence and prescribing for weight management. *Blue Health Intelligence.* May 2024. Accessed September 23, 2024. https://www.bcbs.com/media/pdf/BHI_Issue_Brief_GLP1_Trends.pdf

98. Prillaman M. Obesity drugs aren't always forever. What happens when you quit? *Nature.* 2024;628(8008):488–90.

99. Nelson E. It introduced Ozempic to the world. Now it must remake itself. *The New York Times.* Apr 20, 2024. Accessed September 12, 2024. https://www.nytimes.com/2024/04/20/business/Ozempic-novo-nordisk-wegovy.html

100. Weixel N. Wegovy could bankrupt US health system, Sanders says in new report. *The Hill.* May 15, 2024. Accessed September 12, 2024. https://thehill.com/policy/healthcare/4666461-wegovy-could-bankrupt-u-s-health-system-sanders-says-in-new-report/

101. Levi J, Wang J, Venter F, Hill A. Estimated minimum prices and lowest available national prices for antiobesity medications: improving affordability and access to treatment. *Obesity (Silver Spring).* 2023;31(5):1270–9.

102. Ravinthiran J. Profits over patients. Public Citizen. January 18, 2024. Accessed September 13, 2024. https://www.citizen.org/article/profits-over-patients/

103. DeAngelis CD. Big pharma profits and the public loses. *Milbank Q.* 2016;94(1):30–3.

104. Florko N. Novo Nordisk bought prescribers over 450,000 meals and snacks to promote drugs like Ozempic. StatNews.com. July 5, 2023. Accessed September 13, 2024. https://www.statnews.com/2023/07/05/ozempic-rybelsus-novo-nordisk-meals-for-doctors/

105. Brown C. High price and demand for semaglutide means lack of access for US patients. *BMJ.* 2023;382:1863.

106. Lexchin J, Mintzes B. Semaglutide: a new drug for the treatment of obesity. *DTB.* 2023;61(12):182–8.

107. Real-world trends in GLP-1 treatment persistence and prescribing for weight management. *Blue Health Intelligence.* May 2024. Accessed September 23, 2024. https://www.bcbs.com/media/pdf/BHI_Issue_Brief_GLP1_Trends.pdf

108. Hemo B, Endevelt R, Porath A, Stampfer MJ, Shai I. Adherence to weight loss medications; post-marketing study from HMO pharmacy data of one million individuals. *Diabetes Res Clin Pract.* 2011;94(2):269–75.

109. Ryan DH, Lingvay I, Deanfield J, et al. Long-term weight loss effects of semaglutide in obesity without diabetes in the SELECT trial. *Nat Med.* 2024;30(7):2049–57.

110. Coutinho W, Halpern B. Pharmacotherapy for obesity: moving towards efficacy improvement. *Diabetol Metab Syndr.* 2024;16(1):6.

111. Suran M. As Ozempic's popularity soars, here's what to know about semaglutide and weight loss. *JAMA.* 2023;329(19):1627–9.

112. Smits MM, Holst JJ. Endogenous glucagon-like peptide (GLP)-1 as alternative for GLP-1 receptor agonists: could this work and how? *Diabetes Metab Res Rev.* 2023;39(8):e3699.

113. Suran M. As Ozempic's popularity soars, here's what to know about semaglutide and weight loss. *JAMA.* 2023;329(19):1627–9.

114. Lupianez-Merly C, Dilmaghani S, Vosoughi K, Camilleri M. Review article: Pharmacologic management of obesity—updates on approved medications, indications and risks. *Aliment Pharmacol Ther.* 2024;59(4):475–91.

115. Singh A, Nissen SE. Contemporary management of obesity: a comparison of bariatric metabolic surgery and novel incretin mimetic drugs. *Diabetes Technol Ther.* Published online May 16, 2024.

116. Moyad MA. Embracing the pros and cons of the new weight loss medications (semaglutide, tirzepatide, etc.). *Curr Urol Rep.* 2023;24(11):515–25.

117. U.S. Food and Drug Administration. WEGOVY (semaglutide) injection, for subcutaneous use. FDA.gov. June 2021. Accessed September 13, 2024. https://www.accessdata.fda.gov/drugsatfda_docs/label/2021/215256s000lbl.pdf

118. Lupianez-Merly C, Dilmaghani S, Vosoughi K, Camilleri M. Review article: Pharmacologic management of obesity—updates on approved medications, indications and risks. *Aliment Pharmacol Ther.* 2024;59(4):475–91.

119. Gorgojo-Martínez JJ, Mezquita-Raya P, Carretero-Gómez J, et al. Clinical recommendations to manage gastrointestinal adverse events in patients treated with GLP-1 receptor agonists: a multidisciplinary expert consensus. *J Clin Med.* 2022;12(1):145.

120. Wharton S, Davies M, Dicker D, et al. Managing the gastrointestinal side effects of GLP-1 receptor agonists in obesity: recommendations for clinical practice. *Postgrad Med.* 2022;134(1):14–9.

121. 121 Lupianez-Merly C, Dilmaghani S, Vosoughi K, Camilleri M. Review article: Pharmacologic management of obesity—updates on approved medications, indications and risks. *Aliment Pharmacol Ther.* 2024;59(4):475–91.

122. Kokkorakis M, Katsarou A, Katsiki N, Mantzoros CS. Milestones in the journey towards addressing obesity; past trials and triumphs, recent breakthroughs, and an exciting future in the era of emerging effective medical therapies and integration of effective medical therapies with metabolic surgery. *Metabolism.* 2023;148:155689.

123. Lupianez-Merly C, Dilmaghani S, Vosoughi K, Camilleri M. Review article: Pharmacologic management of obesity—updates on approved medications, indications and risks. *Aliment Pharmacol Ther.* 2024;59(4):475–91.

124. Sen S, Potnuru PP, Hernandez N, et al. Glucagon-like peptide-1 receptor agonist use and residual gastric content before anesthesia. *JAMA Surg.* 2024;159(6):660–7.

125. Jones PM, Hobai IA, Murphy PM. Anesthesia and glucagon-like peptide-1 receptor agonists: proceed with caution! *Can J Anaesth.* 2023;70(8):1281–6.

126. Sen S, Potnuru PP, Hernandez N, et al. Glucagon-like peptide-1 receptor agonist use and residual gastric content before anesthesia. *JAMA Surg.* 2024;159(6):660–7.

127. Locatelli JC, Costa JG, Haynes A, et al. Incretin-based weight loss pharmacotherapy: can resistance exercise optimize changes in body composition? *Diabetes Care.* Published online April 30, 2024:dci230100.

128. Conte C, Hall KD, Klein S. Is weight loss-induced muscle mass loss clinically relevant? *JAMA*. 2024;332(1):9–10.

129. Bikou A, Dermiki-Gkana F, Penteris M, Constantinides TK, Kontogiorgis C. A systematic review of the effect of semaglutide on lean mass: insights from clinical trials. *Expert Opin Pharmacother*. 2024;25(5):611–9.

130. Locatelli JC, Costa JG, Haynes A, et al. Incretin-based weight loss pharmacotherapy: can resistance exercise optimize changes in body composition? *Diabetes Care*. Published online April 30, 2024:dci230100.

131. Locatelli JC, Costa JG, Haynes A, et al. Incretin-based weight loss pharmacotherapy: can resistance exercise optimize changes in body composition? *Diabetes Care*. Published online April 30, 2024:dci230100.

132. Conte C, Hall KD, Klein S. Is weight loss-induced muscle mass loss clinically relevant? *JAMA*. 2024;332(1):9–10.

133. Locatelli JC, Costa JG, Haynes A, et al. Incretin-based weight loss pharmacotherapy: can resistance exercise optimize changes in body composition? *Diabetes Care*. Published online April 30, 2024:dci230100.

134. Conte C, Hall KD, Klein S. Is weight loss-induced muscle mass loss clinically relevant? *JAMA*. 2024;332(1):9–10.

135. Prillaman M. Obesity drugs aren't always forever. What happens when you quit? *Nature*. 2024;628(8008):488–90.

136. Locatelli JC, Costa JG, Haynes A, et al. Incretin-based weight loss pharmacotherapy: can resistance exercise optimize changes in body composition? *Diabetes Care*. Published online April 30, 2024:dci230100.

137. Wang H, He W, Yang G, Zhu L, Liu X. The impact of weight cycling on health and obesity. *Metabolites*. 2024;14(6):344.

138. Locatelli JC, Costa JG, Haynes A, et al. Incretin-based weight loss pharmacotherapy: can resistance exercise optimize changes in body composition? *Diabetes Care*. Published online April 30, 2024:dci230100.

139. Conte C, Hall KD, Klein S. Is weight loss-induced muscle mass loss clinically relevant? *JAMA*. 2024;332(1):9–10.

140. Locatelli JC, Costa JG, Haynes A, et al. Incretin-based weight loss pharmacotherapy: can resistance exercise optimize changes in body composition? *Diabetes Care*. Published online April 30, 2024:dci230100.

141. Sardeli AV, Komatsu TR, Mori MA, Gáspari AF, Chacon-Mikahil MPT. Resistance training prevents muscle loss induced by caloric restriction in obese elderly individuals: a systematic review and meta-analysis. *Nutrients*. 2018;10(4):423.

142. Locatelli JC, Costa JG, Haynes A, et al. Incretin-based weight loss pharmacotherapy: can resistance exercise optimize changes in body composition? *Diabetes Care*. Published online April 30, 2024:dci230100.

143. Carboni A, Woessner S, Martini O, Marroquin NA, Waller J. Natural weight loss or "Ozempic face": demystifying a social media phenomenon. *J Drugs Dermatol*. 2024;23(1):1367–8.

144. O'Neill ES, Wiegmann AL, Parrella N, Pittman T, Hood K, Kurlander D. Injectable weight loss medications in plastic surgery: what we know, perioperative considerations, and recommendations for the future. *Plast Reconstr Surg Glob Open*. 2024;12(1):e5516.

145. Suran M. As Ozempic's popularity soars, here's what to know about semaglutide and weight loss. *JAMA*. 2023;329(19):1627–9.

146. Ridha Z, Fabi SG, Zubair R, Dayan SH. Decoding the implications of glucagon-like peptide-1 receptor agonists on accelerated facial and skin aging. *Aesthet Surg J*. Published online June 14, 2024:sjae132.

147. Haider S, Lipska KJ. Glucagon-like peptide-1 receptor agonists—how safe are they? *JAMA Intern Med*. 2022;182(5):520–1.

148. He L, Wang J, Ping F, et al. Association of glucagon-like peptide-1 receptor agonist use with risk of gallbladder and biliary diseases: a systematic review and meta-analysis of randomized clinical trials. *JAMA Intern Med*. 2022;182(5):513–9.

149. Ruder K. As semaglutide's popularity soars, rare but serious adverse effects are emerging. *JAMA*. 2023;330(22):2140–2.

150. Leehey DJ, Rahman MA, Borys E, Picken MM, Clise CE. Acute kidney injury associated with semaglutide. *Kidney Med*. 2021;3(2):282–5.

151. U.S. Food and Drug Administration. WEGOVY (semaglutide) injection, for subcutaneous use. FDA.gov. June 2021. Accessed September 13, 2024. https://www.accessdata.fda.gov/drugsatfda_docs/label/2021/215256s000lbl.pdf

152. U.S. Food and Drug Administration. ZEPBOUND™ (tirzepatide) injection, for subcutaneous use. FDA.gov. November 2023. Accessed September 13, 2024. https://www.accessdata.fda.gov/drugsatfda_docs/label/2023/217806s000lbl.pdf

153. Silverii GA, Marinelli C, Mannucci E, Rotella F. Glucagon-like peptide-1 receptor agonists and mental health: a meta-analysis of randomized controlled trials. *Diabetes Obes Metab*. 2024;26(6):2505–8.

154. Tang H, Lu Y, Donahoo WT, et al. Glucagon-like peptide-1 receptor agonists and risk for suicidal ideation and behaviors in U. S. older adults with type 2 diabetes: a target trial emulation study. *Ann Intern Med*. 2024;177(8):1004–15.

155. Wang W, Volkow ND, Berger NA, Davis PB, Kaelber DC, Xu R. Association of semaglutide with risk of suicidal ideation in a real-world cohort. *Nat Med*. 2024;30(1):168–76.

156. Bezin J, Gouverneur A, Pénichon M, et al. GLP-1 receptor agonists and the risk of thyroid cancer. *Diabetes Care*. 2023;46(2):384–90.

157. Silverii GA, Monami M, Gallo M, et al. Glucagon-like peptide-1 receptor agonists and risk of thyroid cancer: a systematic review and meta-analysis of randomized controlled trials. *Diabetes Obes Metab*. 2024;26(3):891-900.

158. Silverii GA, Monami M, Gallo M, et al. Glucagon-like peptide-1 receptor agonists and risk of thyroid cancer: a systematic review and meta-analysis of randomized controlled trials. *Diabetes Obes Metab*. 2024;26(3):891-900.

159. National Cancer Institute, Surveillance, Epidemiology, and End Results Program. Cancer stat facts: thyroid cancer. Cancer.gov. Accessed September 13, 2024. https://seer.cancer.gov/statfacts/html/thyro.html

160. National Cancer Institute, Surveillance, Epidemiology, and End Results Program. Cancer stat facts: pancreatic cancer. Cancer.gov. Accessed September 13, 2024. https://seer.cancer.gov/statfacts/html/pancreas.html

161. Sodhi M, Rezaeianzadeh R, Kezouh A, Etminan M. Risk of gastrointestinal adverse events associated with glucagon-like peptide-1 receptor agonists for weight loss. *JAMA*. 2023;330(18):1795–7.

162. Drucker DJ, Holst JJ. The expanding incretin universe: from basic biology to clinical translation. *Diabetologia*. 2023;66(10):1765–79.

163. Kokkorakis M, Katsarou A, Katsiki N, Mantzoros CS. Milestones in the journey towards addressing obesity; past trials and triumphs, recent breakthroughs, and an exciting future in the era of emerging effective medical therapies and integration of effective medical therapies with metabolic surgery. *Metabolism*. 2023;148:155689.

164. Faillie JL, Yin H, Yu OHY, et al. Incretin-based drugs and risk of intestinal obstruction among patients with type 2 diabetes. *Clin Pharmacol Ther*. 2022;111(1):272–82.

165. Sodhi M, Rezaeianzadeh R, Kezouh A, Etminan M. Risk of gastrointestinal adverse events associated with glucagon-like peptide-1 receptor agonists for weight loss. *JAMA*. 2023;330(18):1795–7.

166. Gale E. Incretin therapy: should adverse consequences have been anticipated? *BMJ*. 2013;346:f3617.

167. Butler PC, Elashoff M, Elashoff R, Gale EAM. A critical analysis of the clinical use of incretin-based therapies: are the GLP-1 therapies safe? *Diabetes Care*. 2013;36(7):2118–25.

168. Elashoff M, Matveyenko AV, Gier B, Elashoff R, Butler PC. Pancreatitis, pancreatic, and thyroid cancer with glucagon-like peptide-1-based therapies. *Gastroenterology*. 2011;141(1):150–6.

169. Butler PC, Elashoff M, Elashoff R, Gale EAM. A critical analysis of the clinical use of incretin-based therapies: are the GLP-1 therapies safe? *Diabetes Care*. 2013;36(7):2118–25.

170. Gale EAM. GLP-1 based agents and acute pancreatitis: drug safety falls victim to the three monkey paradigm. *BMJ*. 2013;346:f1263.

171. Butler PC, Elashoff M, Elashoff R, Gale EAM. A critical analysis of the clinical use of incretin-based therapies: are the GLP-1 therapies safe? *Diabetes Care*. 2013;36(7):2118–25.

172. Godlee F. Secrecy does not serve us well. *BMJ*. 2013;346:f3819.

173. Gale E. Incretin therapy: should adverse consequences have been anticipated? *BMJ*. 2013;346:f3617.

174. Godlee F. Secrecy does not serve us well. *BMJ*. 2013;346:f3819.

175. Cohen D. Investigations editor's reply to Holt and to Barnett and O'Hare. *BMJ*. 2013;347:f4383.

176. Gale EAM. GLP-1 based agents and acute pancreatitis: drug safety falls victim to the three monkey paradigm. *BMJ*. 2013;346:f1263.

177. Montori VM. Helping patients make sense of the risks of taking GLP-1 agonists. *BMJ*. 2013;346:f3692.

178. Butler AE, Campbell-Thompson M, Gurlo T, Dawson DW, Atkinson M, Butler PC. Marked expansion of exocrine and endocrine pancreas with incretin therapy in humans with increased exocrine pancreas dysplasia and the potential for glucagon-producing neuroendocrine tumors. *Diabetes*. 2013;62(7):2595–604.

179. Cao M, Pan C, Tian Y, Wang L, Zhao Z, Zhu B. Glucagon-like peptide 1 receptor agonists and the potential risk of pancreatic carcinoma: a pharmacovigilance study using the FDA Adverse Event Reporting System and literature visualization analysis. *Int J Clin Pharm*. 2023;45(3):689–97.

180. Godlee F. Secrecy does not serve us well. *BMJ*. 2013;346:f3819.

181. Asch DA, Luo C, Chen Y. Reports of COVID-19 vaccine adverse events in predominantly Republican vs Democratic states. *JAMA Netw Open*. 2024;7(3):e244177.

182. Hidayat K, Zhou YY, Du HZ, Qin LQ, Shi BM, Li ZN. A systematic review and meta-analysis of observational studies of the association between the use of incretin-based therapies and the risk of pancreatic cancer. *Pharmacoepidemiol Drug Saf*. 2023;32(2):107–25.

183. Cohen D. Has pancreatic damage from glucagon suppressing diabetes drugs been underplayed? *BMJ*. 2013;346:f3680.

184. Recalde M, Pistillo A, Davila-Batista V, et al. Longitudinal body mass index and cancer risk: a cohort study of 2.6 million Catalan adults. *Nat Commun*. 2023;14(1):3816.

185. Wilson RB, Lathigara D, Kaushal D. Systematic review and meta-analysis of the impact of bariatric surgery on future cancer risk. *Int J Mol Sci*. 2023;24(7):6192.

186. Carbonell C, Mathew Stephen M, Ruan Y, Warkentin MT, Brenner DR. Next generation weight loss drugs for the prevention of cancer? *Cancer Control*. 2024;31:10732748241241158.

187. Ahmad FB, Cisewski JA, Anderson RN. Mortality in the United States — provisional data, 2023. *MMWR Morb Mortal Wkly Rep*. 2024;73:677–81.

188. Ryder REJ. The potential risks of pancreatitis and pancreatic cancer with GLP-1-based therapies are far outweighed by the proven and potential (cardiovascular) benefits. *Diabet Med*. 2013;30(10):1148–55.

189. Ruder K. As semaglutide's popularity soars, rare but serious adverse effects are emerging. *JAMA*. 2023;330(22):2140–2.

190. Richards JR, Khalsa SS. Highway to the danger zone? A cautionary account that GLP-1 receptor agonists may be too effective for unmonitored weight loss. *Obes Rev*. 2024;25(5):e13709.

191. Bellini E, Grieco MP, Raposio E. A journey through liposuction and liposculture: review. *Ann Med Surg (Lond)*. 2017;24:53-60.

192. Klein S, Fontana L, Young VL, et al. Absence of an effect of liposuction on insulin action and risk factors for coronary heart disease. *N Engl J Med*. 2004;350(25):2549-57.

193. Blackburn G. Effect of degree of weight loss on health benefits. *Obes Res*. 1995;3 Suppl 2:211s-6s.

194. Klein S, Fontana L, Young VL, et al. Absence of an effect of liposuction on insulin action and risk factors for coronary heart disease. *N Engl J Med*. 2004;350(25):2549-57

195. Scopinaro N. The IFSO and obesity surgery throughout the world. *Obes Surg*. 1998;8(1):3-8.

196. American Society for Metabolic and Bariatric Surgery. Estimate of bariatric surgery numbers, 2011–2022. ASMBS.org. Published 2024. Accessed September 23, 2024. https://asmbs.org/resources/estimate-of-bariatric-surgery-numbers

197. Lupianez-Merly C, Dilmaghani S, Vosoughi K, Camilleri M. Review article: Pharmacologic management of obesity—updates on approved medications, indications and risks. *Aliment Pharmacol Ther*. 2024;59(4):475–91.

198. Kokkorakis M, Katsarou A, Katsiki N, Mantzoros CS. Milestones in the journey towards addressing obesity; past trials and triumphs, recent breakthroughs, and an exciting

future in the era of emerging effective medical therapies and integration of effective medical therapies with metabolic surgery. *Metabolism*. 2023;148:155689.

199. Singh A, Nissen SE. Contemporary management of obesity: a comparison of bariatric metabolic surgery and novel incretin mimetic drugs. *Diabetes Technol Ther*. 2024;26(9):673–85.

200. Singh A, Nissen SE. Contemporary management of obesity: a comparison of bariatric metabolic surgery and novel incretin mimetic drugs. *Diabetes Technol Ther*. 2024;26(9):673–85.

201. Kim MS, Kim JY, Song YS, et al. Association of bariatric surgery with indicated and unintended outcomes: an umbrella review and meta-analysis for risk-benefit assessment. *Obes Rev*. 2024;25(3):e13670.

202. Singh A, Nissen SE. Contemporary management of obesity: a comparison of bariatric metabolic surgery and novel incretin mimetic drugs. *Diabetes Technol Ther*. 2024;26(9):673–85.

203. Abraham J, Butler J, Anker SD. Thinner is better: intentional weight loss and cardiovascular risk. *Med*. 2024;5(4):275–7.

204. Moyad MA. Embracing the pros and cons of the new weight loss medications (semaglutide, tirzepatide, etc.). *Curr Urol Rep*. 2023;24(11):515–25.

205. Lisco G, De Tullio A, Disoteo O, et al. Glucagon-like peptide 1 receptor agonists and thyroid cancer: is it the time to be concerned? *Endocr Connect*. 2023;12(11):e230257.

206. Husain M, Birkenfeld AL, Donsmark M, et al. Oral semaglutide and cardiovascular outcomes in patients with type 2 diabetes. *N Engl J Med*. 2019;381(9):841–51.

207. Kokkorakis M, Katsarou A, Katsiki N, Mantzoros CS. Milestones in the journey towards addressing obesity; past trials and triumphs, recent breakthroughs, and an exciting future in the era of emerging effective medical therapies and integration of effective medical therapies with metabolic surgery. *Metabolism*. 2023;148:155689.

208. Alcido M. Ozempic's main ingredient linked to improved heart health. Forbes.com. May 16, 2024. Accessed September 13, 2024. https://www.forbes.com/health/weight-loss/weight-loss-ozempic-cardiovascular-benefits/

209. Lincoff AM, Brown-Frandsen K, Colhoun HM, et al. Semaglutide and cardiovascular outcomes in obesity without diabetes. *N Engl J Med*. 2023;389(24):2221–32.

210. Lincoff AM, Brown-Frandsen K, Colhoun HM, et al. Semaglutide and cardiovascular outcomes in obesity without diabetes. *N Engl J Med*. 2023;389(24):2221–32.

211. Phizackerley D. Semaglutide reduces the absolute risk of major cardiovascular events by 1.5. *BMJ*. 2024;384:q53.

212. Byrne P, Demasi M, Jones M, Smith SM, O'Brien KK, DuBroff R. Evaluating the association between low-density lipoprotein cholesterol reduction and relative and absolute effects of statin treatment: a systematic review and meta-analysis. *JAMA Intern Med*. 2022;182(5):474–81.

213. U.S. Food and Drug Administration. FDA approves first treatment to reduce risk of serious heart problems specifically in adults with obesity or overweight. FDA.gov. March 8, 2024. Accessed September 13, 2024. https://www.fda.gov/news-events/press-announcements/fda-approves-first-treatment-reduce-risk-serious-heart-problems-specifically-adults-obesity-or

214. Moll H, Frey E, Gerber P, et al. GLP-1 receptor agonists for weight reduction in people living with obesity but without diabetes: a living benefit-harm modelling study. *EClinicalMedicine*. 2024;73:102661.

215. Moll H, Frey E, Gerber P, et al. GLP-1 receptor agonists for weight reduction in people living with obesity but without diabetes: a living benefit-harm modelling study. *EClinicalMedicine*. 2024;73:102661.

216. Hampl SE, Hassink SG, Skinner AC, et al. Clinical practice guideline for the evaluation and treatment of children and adolescents with obesity. *Pediatrics*. 2023;151(2):e2022060640.

217. Klitzman R, Greenberg H. Anti-obesity medications: ethical, policy, and public health concerns. *Hastings Cent Rep*. 2024;54(3):6–10.

218. Butler PC, Elashoff M, Elashoff R, Gale EAM. A critical analysis of the clinical use of incretin-based therapies: are the GLP-1 therapies safe? *Diabetes Care*. 2013;36(7):2118–25.

219. Butler PC, Elashoff M, Elashoff R, Gale EAM. A critical analysis of the clinical use of incretin-based therapies: are the GLP-1 therapies safe? *Diabetes Care*. 2013;36(7):2118–25.

220. 220 Lupianez-Merly C, Dilmaghani S, Vosoughi K, Camilleri M. Review article: Pharmacologic management of obesity—updates on approved medications, indications and risks. *Aliment Pharmacol Ther*. 2024;59(4):475–91.

221. 221 Long B, Pelletier J, Koyfman A, Bridwell RE. GLP-1 agonists: a review for emergency clinicians. *Am J Emerg Med*. 2024;78:89–94.

222. 222 Long B, Pelletier J, Koyfman A, Bridwell RE. GLP-1 agonists: a review for emergency clinicians. *Am J Emerg Med*. 2024;78:89–94.

223. 223 U.S. Food and Drug Administration. Medications containing semaglutide marketed for type 2 diabetes or weight loss. FDA.gov. January 10, 2024. Accessed September 13, 2024. https://www.fda.gov/drugs/postmarket-drug-safety-information-patients-and-providers/medications-containing-semaglutide-marketed-type-2-diabetes-or-weight-loss

224. 224 U.S. Food and Drug Administration. FDA alerts health care providers, compounders and patients of dosing errors associated with compounded injectable semaglutide products. FDA.gov. July 26, 2024. Accessed September 13, 2024. https://www.fda.gov/drugs/human-drug-compounding/fda-alerts-health-care-providers-compounders-and-patients-dosing-errors-associated-compounded

225. 225 Jones CT. The FDA warned Ozempic users. They don't give a f-ck. *Rolling Stone*. June 8, 2023. Accessed September 13, 2024. https://www.rollingstone.com/culture/culture-features/ozempic-semaglutide-fda-warning-compound-drug-1234766348/

226. Moyad MA. Embracing the pros and cons of the new weight loss medications (semaglutide, tirzepatide, etc.). *Curr Urol Rep*. 2023;24(11):515–25.

227. Hu M, Kong Z, Shi Q, Nie J. Acute effect of high-intensity interval training versus moderate-intensity continuous training on appetite-regulating gut hormones in healthy adults: a systematic review and meta-analysis. *Heliyon*. 2023;9(2):e13129.

228. Warburton DER, Bredin SSD. Health benefits of physical activity: a strengths-based approach. *J Clin Med*. 2019;8(12):2044.

229. Yaribeygi H, Jamialahmadi T, Moallem SA, Sahebkar A. Boosting GLP-1 by natural products. *Adv Exp Med Biol*. 2021;1328:513–22.

230. Smits MM, Holst JJ. Endogenous glucagon-like peptide (GLP)-1 as alternative for GLP-1 receptor agonists: could this work and how? *Diabetes Metab Res Rev*. 2023;39(8):e3699.

231. Smits MM, Holst JJ. Endogenous glucagon-like peptide (GLP)-1 as alternative for GLP-1 receptor agonists: could this work and how? *Diabetes Metab Res Rev.* 2023;39(8):e3699.

232. Holst JJ. Glucagon-like peptide-1: are its roles as endogenous hormone and therapeutic wizard congruent? *J Intern Med.* 2022;291(5):557–73.

233. Smits MM, Holst JJ. Endogenous glucagon-like peptide (GLP)-1 as alternative for GLP-1 receptor agonists: could this work and how? *Diabetes Metab Res Rev.* 2023;39(8):e3699.

234. Moyad MA. Embracing the pros and cons of the new weight loss medications (semaglutide, tirzepatide, etc.). *Curr Urol Rep.* 2023;24(11):515–25.

235. Smits MM, Holst JJ. Endogenous glucagon-like peptide (GLP)-1 as alternative for GLP-1 receptor agonists: could this work and how? *Diabetes Metab Res Rev.* 2023;39(8):e3699.

236. Holst JJ. Glucagon-like peptide-1: are its roles as endogenous hormone and therapeutic wizard congruent? *J Intern Med.* 2022;291(5):557–73.

237. Dowsett GKC, Yeo GSH. Are GLP-1R agonists the long-sought-after panacea for obesity? *Trends Mol Med.* 2023;29(10):777–9.

238. Karhunen LJ, Juvonen KR, Huotari A, Purhonen AK, Herzig KH. Effect of protein, fat, carbohydrate and fibre on gastrointestinal peptide release in humans. *Regul Pept.* 2008;149(1–3):70–8.

239. Smits MM, Holst JJ. Endogenous glucagon-like peptide (GLP)-1 as alternative for GLP-1 receptor agonists: could this work and how? *Diabetes Metab Res Rev.* 2023;39(8):e3699.

240. Müller TD, Finan B, Bloom SR, et al. Glucagon-like peptide 1 (GLP-1). *Mol Metab.* 2019;30:72–130.

241. Smits MM, Holst JJ. Endogenous glucagon-like peptide (GLP)-1 as alternative for GLP-1 receptor agonists: could this work and how? *Diabetes Metab Res Rev.* 2023;39(8):e3699.

242. Gutzwiller JP, Göke B, Drewe J, et al. Glucagon-like peptide-1: a potent regulator of food intake in humans. *Gut.* 1999;44(1):81–6.

243. Mars M, Stafleu A, de Graaf C. Use of satiety peptides in assessing the satiating capacity of foods. *Physiol Behav.* 2012;105(2):483–8.

244. Lim JJ, Poppitt SD. How satiating are the "satiety" peptides: a problem of pharmacology versus physiology in the development of novel foods for regulation of food intake. *Nutrients.* 2019;11(7):1517.

245. Gutzwiller JP, Göke B, Drewe J, et al. Glucagon-like peptide-1: a potent regulator of food intake in humans. *Gut.* 1999;44(1):81–6.

246. Li J, Zhang N, Hu L, et al. Improvement in chewing activity reduces energy intake in one meal and modulates plasma gut hormone concentrations in obese and lean young Chinese men. *Am J Clin Nutr.* 2011;94(3):709–16.

247. Kamemoto K, Tataka Y, Hiratsu A, et al. Effect of vegetable consumption with chewing on postprandial glucose metabolism in healthy young men: a randomised controlled study. *Sci Rep.* 2024;14(1):7557.

248. Kokkinos A, le Roux CW, Alexiadou K, et al. Eating slowly increases the postprandial response of the anorexigenic gut hormones, peptide YY and glucagon-like peptide-1. *J Clin Endocrinol Metab.* 2010;95(1):333–7.

249. Okrent A, Sweitzer M, Young S, Page ET. Researchers adjust self-reported estimates of obesity in scanner data. USDA Economic Research Service. November 20, 2023. Accessed September 14, 2024. https://www.ers.usda.gov/amber-waves/2023/november/researchers-adjust-self-reported-estimates-of-obesity-in-scanner-data/

250. Rigamonti AE, Agosti F, Compri E, et al. Anorexigenic postprandial responses of PYY and GLP1 to slow ice cream consumption: preservation in obese adolescents, but not in obese adults. *Eur J Endocrinol*. 2013;168(3):429–36.

251. Yaribeygi H, Jamialahmadi T, Moallem SA, Sahebkar A. Boosting GLP-1 by natural products. *Adv Exp Med Biol*. 2021;1328:513–22.

252. Watanabe K, Igarashi M, Li X, et al. Dietary soybean protein ameliorates high-fat diet-induced obesity by modifying the gut microbiota-dependent biotransformation of bile acids. *PLoS One*. 2018;13(8):e0202083.

253. Mietlicki-Baase EG, Koch-Laskowski K, McGrath LE, et al. Daily supplementation of dietary protein improves the metabolic effects of GLP-1-based pharmacotherapy in lean and obese rats. *Physiol Behav*. 2017;177:122–8.

254. Park S, Ahn IS, Kim JH, Lee MR, Kim JS, Kim HJ. Glyceollins, one of the phytoalexins derived from soybeans under fungal stress, enhance insulin sensitivity and exert insulinotropic actions. *J Agric Food Chem*. 2010;58(3):1551–7.

255. Liu C, Hu MY, Zhang M, et al. Association of GLP-1 secretion with anti-hyperlipidemic effect of ginsenosides in high-fat diet fed rats. *Metabolism*. 2014;63(10):1342–51.

256. Wang HP, Lin ZZ, Yin Q, Du J. Screening of GLP-1r agonists from natural products using affinity ultrafiltration screening coupled with UPLC-ESI-Orbitrap-MS technology: a case study of Panax ginseng. *J Asian Nat Prod Res*. Published online July 22, 2024:1–13.

257. Yaribeygi H, Jamialahmadi T, Moallem SA, Sahebkar A. Boosting GLP-1 by natural products. *Adv Exp Med Biol*. 2021;1328:513–22.

258. Shin JS, Huh YS. Effect of intake of gardenia fruits and combined exercise of middle-aged obese women on hormones regulating energy metabolism. *J Exerc Nutrition Biochem*. 2014;18(1):41–9.

259. Pegah A, Abbasi-Oshaghi E, Khodadadi I, Mirzaei F, Tayebinai H. Probiotic and resveratrol normalize GLP-1 levels and oxidative stress in the intestine of diabetic rats. *Metabol Open*. 2021;10:100093.

260. Thazhath SS, Wu T, Bound MJ, et al. Administration of resveratrol for 5 wk has no effect on glucagon-like peptide 1 secretion, gastric emptying, or glycemic control in type 2 diabetes: a randomized controlled trial. *Am J Clin Nutr*. 2016;103(1):66–70.

261. Liu CY, Huang CJ, Huang LH, Chen IJ, Chiu JP, Hsu CH. Effects of green tea extract on insulin resistance and glucagon-like peptide 1 in patients with type 2 diabetes and lipid abnormalities: a randomized, double-blinded, and placebo-controlled trial. *PLoS One*. 2014;9(3):e91163.

262. Thomsen C, Rasmussen O, Lousen T, et al. Differential effects of saturated and monounsaturated fatty acids on postprandial lipemia and incretin responses in healthy subjects. *Am J Clin Nutr*. 1999;69(6):1135–43.

263. Thomsen C, Storm H, Holst JJ, Hermansen K. Differential effects of saturated and monounsaturated fats on postprandial lipemia and glucagon-like peptide 1 responses in patients with type 2 diabetes. *Am J Clin Nutr*. 2003;77(3):605–1.

264. Seery C. Eating avocados as effective as weight loss injections, expert claims. Diabetes.co.uk. June 20, 2023. Accessed September 14, 2024. https://www.diabetes.co.uk/news/2023/jun/eating-avocados-as-effective-as-weight-loss-injections-expert-claims.html

265. Stearn E. I'm a nutritionist—these are the foods that work just like miracle weight loss jab Ozempic. DailyMail.com. June 9, 2023. Accessed September 14, 2024. https://www.dailymail.co.uk/health/article-12176793/Im-nutritionist-foods-work-just-like-miracle-weight-loss-jab-Ozempic.html

266. Corella-Salazar DA, Domínguez-Avila JA, Montiel-Herrera M, et al. Sub-chronic consumption of a phenolic-rich avocado paste extract induces GLP-1-, leptin-, and adiponectin-mediated satiety in Wistar rats. *J Food Biochem*. 2021;45(11):e13957.

267. Haddad E, Wien M, Oda K, Sabaté J. Postprandial gut hormone responses to Hass avocado meals and their association with visual analog scores in overweight adults: a randomized 3 × 3 crossover trial. *Eat Behav*. 2018;31:35–40.

268. Henderson J. What to know about berberine, the supplement dubbed 'nature's Ozempic.' ABC News. June 15, 2023. Accessed September 14, 2024. https://abcnews.go.com/GMA/Wellness/berberine-supplement-viral-social-media-natures-ozempic/story?id=99867653

269. Greger M. Treating acne with barberries. NutritionFacts.org. February 5, 2016. Accessed September 14, 2024. https://nutritionfacts.org/video/treating-acne-barberries/

270. Yu Y, Liu L, Wang X, et al. Modulation of glucagon-like peptide-1 release by berberine: *in vivo* and *in vitro* studies. *Biochem Pharmacol*. 2010;79(7):1000–6.

271. Amini MR, Sheikhhossein F, Naghshi S, et al. Effects of berberine and barberry on anthropometric measures: a systematic review and meta-analysis of randomized controlled trials. *Complement Ther Med*. 2020;49:102337.

272. King K, Lin NP, Cheng YH, Chen GH, Chein RJ. Isolation of positive modulator of glucagon-like peptide-1 signaling from *trigonella foenum-graecum* (fenugreek) seed. *J Biol Chem*. 2015;290(43):26235–48.

273. Chou IW, Cheng YH, Chen YR, Hsieh PCH, King K. Fenugreek compound (N55) lowers plasma glucose through the enhancement of response of physiological glucagon-like peptide-1. *Sci Rep*. 2017;7(1):12265.

274. Haldar S, Chia SC, Henry CJ. Polyphenol-rich curry made with mixed spices and vegetables increases postprandial plasma GLP-1 concentration in a dose-dependent manner. *Eur J Clin Nutr*. 2018;72(2):297–300.

275. Samad MB, Mohsin MNAB, Razu BA, et al. [6]-Gingerol, from *Zingiber officinale*, potentiates GLP-1 mediated glucose-stimulated insulin secretion pathway in pancreatic β-cells and increases RAB8/RAB10-regulated membrane presentation of GLUT4 transporters in skeletal muscle to improve hyperglycemia in Leprdb/db type 2 diabetic mice. *BMC Complement Altern Med*. 2017;17(1):395.

276. Al Asoom L, Alassaf MA, AlSulaiman NS, et al. The effectiveness of *Nigella sativa* and ginger as appetite suppressants: an experimental study on healthy Wistar rats. *Vasc Health Risk Manag*. 2023;19:1–11.

277. Hu ML, Rayner CK, Wu KL, et al. Effect of ginger on gastric motility and symptoms of functional dyspepsia. *World J Gastroenterol*. 2011;17(1):105–10.

278. Sharma P, Joshi T, Joshi T, Chandra S, Tamta S. *In silico* screening of potential antidiabetic phytochemicals from *Phyllanthus emblica* against therapeutic targets of type 2 diabetes. *J Ethnopharmacol*. 2020;248:112268.

279. Thota RN, Dias CB, Abbott KA, Acharya SH, Garg ML. Curcumin alleviates postprandial glycaemic response in healthy subjects: a cross-over, randomized controlled study. *Sci Rep*. 2018;8(1):13679.

280. Takikawa M, Kurimoto Y, Tsuda T. Curcumin stimulates glucagon-like peptide-1 secretion in GLUTag cells via Ca2+/calmodulin-dependent kinase II activation. *Biochem Biophys Res Commun.* 2013;435(2):165–70.

281. He Y, Chen X, Li Y, et al. Curcumin supplementation alleviates hepatic fat content associated with modulation of gut microbiota-dependent bile acid metabolism in patients with nonalcoholic simple fatty liver disease: a randomized controlled trial. *Am J Clin Nutr.* 2024;120(1):66–79.

282. Dehzad MJ, Ghalandari H, Nouri M, Askarpour M. Effects of curcumin/turmeric supplementation on obesity indices and adipokines in adults: a grade-assessed systematic review and dose-response meta-analysis of randomized controlled trials. *Phytother Res.* 2023;37(4):1703-28.

283. Hlebowicz J, Hlebowicz A, Lindstedt S, et al. Effects of 1 and 3 g cinnamon on gastric emptying, satiety, and postprandial blood glucose, insulin, glucose-dependent insulinotropic polypeptide, glucagon-like peptide 1, and ghrelin concentrations in healthy subjects. *Am J Clin Nutr.* 2009;89(3):815–21.

284. Keramati M, Musazadeh V, Malekahmadi M, et al. Cinnamon, an effective anti-obesity agent: evidence from an umbrella meta-analysis. *J Food Biochem.* 2022;46(8):e14166.

285. Smeets AJ, Westerterp-Plantenga MS. The acute effects of a lunch containing capsaicin on energy and substrate utilisation, hormones, and satiety. *Eur J Nutr.* 2009;48(4):229–34.

286. Zhang W, Zhang Q, Wang L, et al. The effects of capsaicin intake on weight loss among overweight and obese subjects: a systematic review and meta-analysis of randomised controlled trials. *Br J Nutr.* 2023;130(9):1645–56.

287. Zuluaga G. Potential of bitter medicinal plants: a review of flavor physiology. *Pharmaceuticals (Basel).* 2024;17(6):722.

288. Walker EG, Lo KR, Pahl MC, et al. An extract of hops (*Humulus lupulus* L.) modulates gut peptide hormone secretion and reduces energy intake in healthy-weight men: a randomized, crossover clinical trial. *Am J Clin Nutr.* 2022;115(3):925–40.

289. Latorre R, Huynh J, Mazzoni M, et al. Expression of the bitter taste receptor, T2R38, in enteroendocrine cells of the colonic mucosa of overweight/obese vs. lean subjects. *PLoS One.* 2016;11(2):e0147468.

290. Rezaie P, Bitarafan V, Rose BD, et al. Quinine effects on gut and pancreatic hormones and antropyloroduodenal pressures in humans—role of delivery site and sex. *J Clin Endocrinol Metab.* 2022;107(7):e2870–81.

291. Walker EG, Lo KR, Pahl MC, et al. An extract of hops (*Humulus lupulus* L.) modulates gut peptide hormone secretion and reduces energy intake in healthy-weight men: a randomized, crossover clinical trial. *Am J Clin Nutr.* 2022;115(3):925–40.

292. Walker E, Lo K, Tham S, et al. New Zealand bitter hops extract reduces hunger during a 24 h water only fast. *Nutrients.* 2019;11(11):2754.

293. Walker EG, Lo KR, Pahl MC, et al. An extract of hops (*Humulus lupulus* L.) modulates gut peptide hormone secretion and reduces energy intake in healthy-weight men: a randomized, crossover clinical trial. *Am J Clin Nutr.* 2022;115(3):925–40.

294. Nasri A, Pohjanvirta R. Comparison of *in vitro* toxicities of 8-prenylnaringenin, tartrazine and 17β-estradiol, representatives of natural and synthetic estrogens, in rat and human hepatoma cell lines. *Endocr Res.* 2024;49(2):106–16.

295. For more, see *What Are the Effects of the Hops Phytoestrogen in Beer?* at see.nf/hops.

296. Ferrari P, Licaj I, Muller DC, et al. Lifetime alcohol use and overall and cause-specific mortality in the European Prospective Investigation into Cancer and nutrition (EPIC) study. *BMJOpen*. 2014;4:e005245.

297. Park SH, Hoang T, Kim J. Dietary factors and breast cancer prognosis among breast cancer survivors: a systematic review and meta-analysis of cohort studies. *Cancers (Basel)*. 2021;13(21):5329.

298. Rezaie P, Bitarafan V, Rose BD, et al. Quinine effects on gut and pancreatic hormones and antropyloroduodenal pressures in humans—role of delivery site and sex. *J Clin Endocrinol Metab*. 2022;107(7):e2870–81.

299. George JN, Morton JM, Liles NW, Nester CM. After the party's over. *N Engl J Med*. 2017;376(1):74–80.

300. Bitarafan V, Fitzgerald PCE, Little TJ, et al. Intragastric administration of the bitter tastant quinine lowers the glycemic response to a nutrient drink without slowing gastric emptying in healthy men. *Am J Physiol Regul Integr Comp Physiol*. 2020;318(2):R263–73.

301. Heybach JP, Boyle PC. Dietary quinine reduces body weight and food intake independent of aversive taste. *Physiol Behav*. 1982;29(6):1171–3.

302. Iven J, Biesiekierski JR, Zhao D, et al. Intragastric quinine administration decreases hedonic eating in healthy women through peptide-mediated gut-brain signaling mechanisms. *Nutr Neurosci*. 2019;22(12):850–62.

303. Saguil A, Lauters R. Quinine for leg cramps. *Am Fam Physician*. 2016;93(3):177–8.

304. Federal Institute for Risk Assessment. Quinine-containing beverages may cause health problems. BfR. February 17, 2005. Updated May 9, 2008. Accessed September 14, 2024. https://www.bfr.bund.de/cm/349/quinine_containing_beverages_may_cause_health_problems.pdf

305. Andreozzi P, Sarnelli G, Pesce M, et al. The bitter taste receptor agonist quinine reduces calorie intake and increases the postprandial release of cholecystokinin in healthy subjects. *J Neurogastroenterol Motil*. 2015;21(4):511–9.

306. U.S. Department of Agriculture, Agricultural Research Service. Beverages, carbonated, tonic water. FoodData Central. April 1, 2019. Accessed September 14, 2024. https://fdc.nal.usda.gov/fdc-app.html?query=tonic+water&utf8=%E2%9C%93&affili#/food-details/171869/nutrients

307. Chiurazzi M, De Conno B, Di Lauro M, et al. The effects of a cinchona supplementation on satiety, weight loss and body composition in a population of overweight/obese adults: a controlled randomized study. *Nutrients*. 2023;15(24):5033.

308. Andreozzi P, Sarnelli G, Pesce M, et al. The bitter taste receptor agonist quinine reduces calorie intake and increases the postprandial release of cholecystokinin in healthy subjects. *J Neurogastroenterol Motil*. 2015;21(4):511–9.

309. Chiurazzi M, De Conno B, Di Lauro M, et al. The effects of a cinchona supplementation on satiety, weight loss and body composition in a population of overweight/obese adults: a controlled randomized study. *Nutrients*. 2023;15(24):5033.

310. Liles NW, Page EE, Liles AL, Vesely SK, Raskob GE, George JN. Diversity and severity of adverse reactions to quinine: a systematic review. *Am J Hematol*. 2016;91(5):461–6.

311. Brasić JR. Should people with nocturnal leg cramps drink tonic water and bitter lemon? *Psychol Rep*. 1999;84(2):355–67.

312. Howard MA, Hibbard AB, Terrell DR, Medina PJ, Vesely SK, George JN. Quinine allergy causing acute severe systemic illness: report of 4 patients manifesting multiple hematologic, renal, and hepatic abnormalities. *Proc (Bayl Univ Med Cent).* 2003;16(1):21–6.

313. Liles NW, Page EE, Liles AL, Vesely SK, Raskob GE, George JN. Diversity and severity of adverse reactions to quinine: a systematic review. *Am J Hematol.* 2016;91(5):461–6.

314. Bohne AS, Dietrich C, Morrison K, Schwarz T, Wehkamp U, Kaeding M. Two cases of quinine-induced fixed "drug" eruption induced by long drinks. *J Eur Acad Dermatol Venereol.* 2021;35(11):e774–6.

315. Lonsdale-Eccles E, Wallett A, Ward AM. A case of fixed drug eruption secondary to quinine in tonic water presenting to a sexual health clinic. *Sex Transm Infect.* 2014;90(5):356–7.

316. Wada S, Namiki T, Tokoro S, Miura K, Yokozeki H. Stevens-Johnson syndrome induced by tonic water. *J Eur Acad Dermatol Venereol.* 2021;35(10):e662–3.

317. Liles NW, Page EE, Liles AL, Vesely SK, Raskob GE, George JN. Diversity and severity of adverse reactions to quinine: a systematic review. *Am J Hematol.* 2016;91(5):461–6.

318. Gelfman DM. Reflections on quinine and its importance in dermatology today. *Clin Dermatol.* 2021;39(5):900–3.

319. Osinubi AA, Noronha CC, Okanlawon AO. Morphometric and stereological assessment of the effects of long-term administration of quinine on the morphology of rat testis. *West Afr J Med.* 2005;24(3):200–5.

320. Taylor S. Quinine intoxications: a continuing problem. *Br J Clin Pharmacol.* 2004;57(6):817; author reply 817.

321. Bacon P, Spalton DJ, Smith SE. Blindness from quinine toxicity. *Br J Ophthalmol.* 1988;72(3):219–24.

322. Traill A. Quinine iris toxicity. *Arch Ophthalmol.* 2007;125(3):430.

323. El-Tawil S, Al Musa T, Valli H, et al. Quinine for muscle cramps. *Cochrane Database Syst Rev.* 2015;2015(4):CD005044.

324. Brasić JR. Risks of the consumption of beverages containing quinine. *Psychol Rep.* 2003;93(3 Pt 2):1022–4.

325. U.S. Food and Drug Administration. Drug products containing quinine; enforcement action dates. Docket no. 2006N-0476. FederalRegister.gov. December 15, 2006. Accessed September 14, 2024. https://www.federalregister.gov/documents/2006/12/15/06-9713/drug-products-containing-quinine-enforcement-action-dates

326. U.S. Food and Drug Administration. Serious risks associated with using Quinine to prevent or treat nocturnal leg cramps. FDA.gov. September 2012. Accessed September 14, 2024. https://www.fda.gov/files/about%20fda/published/Serious-risks-associated-with-using-Quinine-to-prevent-or-treat-nocturnal-leg-cramps.pdf

327. Taylor S. Quinine intoxications: a continuing problem. *Br J Clin Pharmacol.* 2004;57(6):817; author reply 817.

328. Moshirfar M, Somani SN, Shmunes KM, Ronquillo YC. Will tonic water stop my eyelid twitching? *Clin Ophthalmol.* 2020;14:689–91.

329. Brasić JR. Risks of the consumption of beverages containing quinine. *Psychol Rep.* 2003;93(3 Pt 2):1022–4.

330. Worden AN, Frape DL, Shephard NW. Consumption of quinine hydrochloride in tonic water. *Lancet*. 1987;1(8527):271–2.

331. Berglund F. Toxicity of quinine. *Toxicology*. 1989;58(3):237–8.

332. Brasić JR. Should people with nocturnal leg cramps drink tonic water and bitter lemon? *Psychol Rep*. 1999;84(2):355–67.

333. Horgan SE, Williams RW. Chronic retinal toxicity due to quinine in Indian tonic water. *Eye (Lond)*. 1995;9(Pt 5):637–8.

334. Elmusa E, Asghar H, Hamza A, Raza MW, Rodriguez I. Quinine water-triggered atrial tachyarrhythmia. *Cureus*. 2022;14(12):e32706.

335. Drewitt PN, Butterworth KR, Springall CD, Walters DG, Raglan EM. Toxicity threshold of quinine hydrochloride following low-level repeated dosing in healthy volunteers. *Food Chem Toxicol*. 1993;31(4):235–45.

336. Colley JC, Edwards JA, Heywood R, Purser D. Toxicity studies with quinine hydrochloride. *Toxicology*. 1989;54(2):219–26.

337. Duncan ADS, Hapca S, De Souza N, Morales D, Bell S. Quinine exposure and the risk of acute kidney injury: a population-based observational study of older people. *Age Ageing*. 2020;49(6):1042–7.

338. Fardet L, Nazareth I, Petersen I. Association between long-term quinine exposure and all-cause mortality. *JAMA*. 2017;317(18):1907–9.

339. Brasić JR. Risks of the consumption of beverages containing quinine. *Psychol Rep*. 2003;93(3 Pt 2):1022–4.

340. Ohira A, Yamaguchi S, Miyagi T, et al. Fixed eruption due to quinine in tonic water: a case report with high-performance liquid chromatography and ultraviolet A analyses. *J Dermatol*. 2013;40(8):629–31.

341. Marques JG, Calado G, Martins P, Pinto PL. Tonic water: a rare cause of exanthema. *Allergol Immunopathol (Madr)*. 2012;40(1):60–1.

342. Huang RY, Huang CC, Hu FB, Chavarro JE. Vegetarian diets and weight reduction: a meta-analysis of randomized controlled trials. *J Gen Intern Med*. 2016;31(1):109–16.

343. Belinova L, Kahleova H, Malinska H, et al. Differential acute postprandial effects of processed meat and isocaloric vegan meals on the gastrointestinal hormone response in subjects suffering from type 2 diabetes and healthy controls: a randomized crossover study. *PLoS One*. 2014;9(9):e107561.

344. Kahleova H, Tura A, Klementova M, et al. A plant-based meal stimulates incretin and insulin secretion more than an energy- and macronutrient-matched standard meal in type 2 diabetes: a randomized crossover study. *Nutrients*. 2019;11(3):486.

345. Kahleova H, Tintera J, Thieme L, et al. A plant-based meal affects thalamus perfusion differently than an energy- and macronutrient-matched conventional meal in men with type 2 diabetes, overweight/obese, and healthy men: a three-group randomized crossover study. *Clin Nutr*. 2021;40(4):1822–33.

346. Klementova M, Thieme L, Haluzik M, et al. A plant-based meal increases gastrointestinal hormones and satiety more than an energy- and macronutrient-matched processed-meat meal in T2D, obese, and healthy men: a three-group randomized crossover study. *Nutrients*. 2019;11(1):157.

347. Muhlhausler BS, Belobrajdic D, Wymond B, Benassi-Evans B. Assessing the effect of plant-based mince on fullness and post-prandial satiety in healthy male subjects. *Nutrients*. 2022;14(24):5326.

348. Huang RY, Huang CC, Hu FB, Chavarro JE. Vegetarian diets and weight reduction: a meta-analysis of randomized controlled trials. *J Gen Intern Med*. 2016;31(1):109–16.

349. Cherta-Murillo A, Lett AM, Frampton J, Chambers ES, Finnigan TJA, Frost GS. Effects of mycoprotein on glycaemic control and energy intake in humans: a systematic review. *Br J Nutr*. 2020;123(12):1321–2.

350. Wright N, Wilson L, Smith M, Duncan B, McHugh P. The BROAD study: a randomised controlled trial using a whole food plant-based diet in the community for obesity, ischaemic heart disease or diabetes. *Nutr Diabetes*. 2017;7(3):e256.

351. Ivanova S, Delattre C, Karcheva-Bahchevanska D, Benbasat N, Nalbantova V, Ivanov K. Plant-based diet as a strategy for weight control. *Foods*. 2021;10(12):3052.

352. Kamakura R, Raza GS, Sodum N, Lehto VP, Kovalainen M, Herzig KH. Colonic delivery of nutrients for sustained and prolonged release of gut peptides: a novel strategy for appetite management. *Mol Nutr Food Res*. 2022;66(19):e2200192.

353. Drucker DJ, Holst JJ. The expanding incretin universe: from basic biology to clinical translation. *Diabetologia*. 2023;66(10):1765–79.

354. Kamakura R, Raza GS, Sodum N, Lehto VP, Kovalainen M, Herzig KH. Colonic delivery of nutrients for sustained and prolonged release of gut peptides: a novel strategy for appetite management. *Mol Nutr Food Res*. 2022;66(19):e2200192.

355. I discuss the ileal brake in detail in my *Evidence-Based Weight Loss* presentation at see.nf/weight.

356. van Avesaat M, Troost FJ, Ripken D, Hendriks HF, Masclee AAM. Ileal brake activation: macronutrient-specific effects on eating behavior? *Int J Obes (Lond)*. 2015;39(2):235–43.

357. Karhunen LJ, Juvonen KR, Huotari A, Purhonen AK, Herzig KH. Effect of protein, fat, carbohydrate and fibre on gastrointestinal peptide release in humans. *Regul Pept*. 2008;149(1-3):70–8.

358. van Avesaat M, Troost FJ, Ripken D, Hendriks HF, Masclee AAM. Ileal brake activation: macronutrient-specific effects on eating behavior? *Int J Obes (Lond)*. 2015;39(2):235–43.

359. Qin W, Ying W, Hamaker B, Zhang G. Slow digestion-oriented dietary strategy to sustain the secretion of GLP-1 for improved glucose homeostasis. *Compr Rev Food Sci Food Saf*. 2021;20(5):5173–96.

360. Jenkins DJ, Kendall CW. The Garden of Eden: plant-based diets, the genetic drive to store fat and conserve cholesterol, and implications for epidemiology in the 21st century. *Epidemiology*. 2006;17(2):128–30.

361. Rubio-Ruiz ME, Peredo-Escárcega AE, Cano-Martínez A, Guarner-Lans V. An evolutionary perspective of nutrition and inflammation as mechanisms of cardiovascular disease. *Int J Evol Biol*. 2015;2015:179791.

362. Eaton SB, Konner M. Paleolithic nutrition. A consideration of its nature and current implications. *N Engl J Med*. 1985;312(5):283–9.

363. Anderson JW, Konz EC, Jenkins DJ. Health advantages and disadvantages of weight-reducing diets: a computer analysis and critical review. *J Am Coll Nutr*. 2000;19(5):578–90.

364. Kamakura R, Raza GS, Sodum N, Lehto VP, Kovalainen M, Herzig KH. Colonic delivery of nutrients for sustained and prolonged release of gut peptides: a novel strategy for appetite management. *Mol Nutr Food Res*. 2022;66(19):e2200192.

365. Grassby T, Picout DR, Mandalari G, et al. Modelling of nutrient bioaccessibility in almond seeds based on the fracture properties of their cell walls. *Food Funct.* 2014;5(12):3096–106.

366. Kamakura R, Raza GS, Sodum N, Lehto VP, Kovalainen M, Herzig KH. Colonic delivery of nutrients for sustained and prolonged release of gut peptides: a novel strategy for appetite management. *Mol Nutr Food Res.* 2022;66(19):e2200192.

367. Levine AS, Silvis SE. Absorption of whole peanuts, peanut oil, and peanut butter. *N Engl J Med.* 1980;303(16):917–8.

368. Qin W, Ying W, Hamaker B, Zhang G. Slow digestion-oriented dietary strategy to sustain the secretion of GLP-1 for improved glucose homeostasis. *Compr Rev Food Sci Food Saf.* 2021;20(5):5173–96.

369. Reimann F. Dorothy Hodgkin lecture 2023: The enteroendocrine system—sensors in your guts. *Diabet Med.* 2023;40(12):e15212.

370. Qin W, Ying W, Hamaker B, Zhang G. Slow digestion-oriented dietary strategy to sustain the secretion of GLP-1 for improved glucose homeostasis. *Compr Rev Food Sci Food Saf.* 2021;20(5):5173–96.

371. Eaton SB, Eaton III SB, Konner MJ. Paleolithic nutrition revisited: a twelve-year retrospective on its nature and implications. *Eur J Clin Nutr.* 1997;51(4):207–16.

372. U.S. Department of Agriculture, Agricultural Research Service. Nutrient intakes from food and beverages: mean amounts consumed per individual, by gender and age, What We Eat in America, NHANES 2017-March 2020 prepandemic. 2022. Accessed September 23, 2024. https://www.ars.usda.gov/ARSUserFiles/80400530/pdf/1720/Table_1_NIN_GEN_1720.pdf

373. Kahleova H, Tintera J, Thieme L, et al. A plant-based meal affects thalamus perfusion differently than an energy- and macronutrient-matched conventional meal in men with type 2 diabetes, overweight/obese, and healthy men: a three-group randomized crossover study. *Clin Nutr.* 2021;40(4):1822–33.

374. McCarty MF, DiNicolantonio JJ. Acarbose, lente carbohydrate, and prebiotics promote metabolic health and longevity by stimulating intestinal production of GLP-1. *Open Heart.* 2015;2(1):e000205.

375. Kamakura R, Raza GS, Sodum N, Lehto VP, Kovalainen M, Herzig KH. Colonic delivery of nutrients for sustained and prolonged release of gut peptides: a novel strategy for appetite management. *Mol Nutr Food Res.* 2022;66(19):e2200192.

376. Schmidt JA, Rinaldi S, Scalbert A, et al. Plasma concentrations and intakes of amino acids in male meat-eaters, fish-eaters, vegetarians and vegans: a cross-sectional analysis in the EPIC-Oxford cohort. *Eur J Clin Nutr.* 2016;70(3):306–12.

377. Angelini G, Russo S, Mingrone G. Incretin hormones, obesity and gut microbiota. *Peptides.* 2024;178:171216.

378. Müller M, Hernández MAG, Goossens GH, et al. Circulating but not faecal short-chain fatty acids are related to insulin sensitivity, lipolysis and GLP-1 concentrations in humans. *Sci Rep.* 2019;9(1):12515.

379. Freeland KR, Wolever TMS. Acute effects of intravenous and rectal acetate on glucagon-like peptide-1, peptide YY, ghrelin, adiponectin and tumour necrosis factor-alpha. *Br J Nutr.* 2010;103(3):460–6.

380. Bridges SR, Anderson JW, Deakins DA, Dillon DW, Wood CL. Oat bran increases serum acetate of hypercholesterolemic men. *Am J Clin Nutr.* 1992;56(2):455–9.

381. Hernández MAG, Canfora EE, Jocken JWE, Blaak EE. The short-chain fatty acid acetate in body weight control and insulin sensitivity. *Nutrients*. 2019;11(8):1943.

382. Ali Z, Wang Z, Amir RM, et al. Potential uses of vinegar as a medicine and related *in vivo* mechanisms. *Int J Vitam Nutr Res*. 2018;86(3–4):1–12.

383. Byrne CS, Chambers ES, Alhabeeb H, et al. Increased colonic propionate reduces anticipatory reward responses in the human striatum to high-energy foods. *Am J Clin Nutr*. 2016;104(1):5–14.

384. Smits MM, Holst JJ. Endogenous glucagon-like peptide (GLP)-1 as alternative for GLP-1 receptor agonists: could this work and how? *Diabetes Metab Res Rev*. 2023;39(8):e3699.

385. Chambers ES, Viardot A, Psichas A, et al. Effects of targeted delivery of propionate to the human colon on appetite regulation, body weight maintenance and adiposity in overweight adults. *Gut*. 2015;64(11):1744–54.

386. Piche T, des Varannes SB, Sacher-Huvelin S, Holst JJ, Cuber JC, Galmiche JP. Colonic fermentation influences lower esophageal sphincter function in gastroesophageal reflux disease. *Gastroenterology*. 2003;124(4):894–902.

387. Cani PD, Lecourt E, Dewulf EM, et al. Gut microbiota fermentation of prebiotics increases satietogenic and incretin gut peptide production with consequences for appetite sensation and glucose response after a meal. *Am J Clin Nutr*. 2009;90(5):1236–43.

388. Zeng Y, Wu Y, Zhang Q, Xiao X. Crosstalk between glucagon-like peptide 1 and gut microbiota in metabolic diseases. *mBio*. 2024;15(1):e0203223.

389. Kabisch S, Weickert MO, Pfeiffer AFH. The role of cereal soluble fiber in the beneficial modulation of glycometabolic gastrointestinal hormones. *Crit Rev Food Sci Nutr*. 2024;64(13):4331–47.

390. Karhunen LJ, Juvonen KR, Huotari A, Purhonen AK, Herzig KH. Effect of protein, fat, carbohydrate and fibre on gastrointestinal peptide release in humans. *Regul Pept*. 2008;149(1-3):70–8.

391. Akhlaghi M. The role of dietary fibers in regulating appetite, an overview of mechanisms and weight consequences. *Crit Rev Food Sci Nutr*. 2024;64(10):3139–50.

392. Kabisch S, Weickert MO, Pfeiffer AFH. The role of cereal soluble fiber in the beneficial modulation of glycometabolic gastrointestinal hormones. *Crit Rev Food Sci Nutr*. 2024;64(13):4331–47.

393. Santaliestra-Pasías AM, Garcia-Lacarte M, Rico MC, Aguilera CM, Moreno LA. Effect of two bakery products on short-term food intake and gut-hormones in young adults: a pilot study. *Int J Food Sci Nutr*. 2015;67(5):562–70.

394. Ye Z, Arumugam V, Haugabrooks E, Williamson P, Hendrich S. Soluble dietary fiber (Fibersol-2) decreased hunger and increased satiety hormones in humans when ingested with a meal. *Nutr Res*. 2015;35(5):393–400.

395. Santaliestra-Pasías AM, Garcia-Lacarte M, Rico MC, Aguilera CM, Moreno LA. Effect of two bakery products on short-term food intake and gut-hormones in young adults: a pilot study. *Int J Food Sci Nutr*. 2015;67(5):562–70.

396. Qin W, Ying W, Hamaker B, Zhang G. Slow digestion-oriented dietary strategy to sustain the secretion of GLP-1 for improved glucose homeostasis. *Compr Rev Food Sci Food Saf*. 2021;20(5):5173–96.

397. Angelini G, Russo S, Mingrone G. Incretin hormones, obesity and gut microbiota. *Peptides*. 2024;178:171216.

398. Freeland KR, Wilson C, Wolever TMS. Adaptation of colonic fermentation and glucagon-like peptide-1 secretion with increased wheat fibre intake for 1 year in hyperinsulinaemic human subjects. *Br J Nutr*. 2010;103(1):82–90.

399. Hamaker BR, Cantu-Jungles TM. Discrete fiber structures dictate human gut bacteria outcomes. *Trends Endocrinol Metab*. 2020;31(11):803–5.

400. Toribio-Mateas M. Harnessing the power of microbiome assessment tools as part of neuroprotective nutrition and lifestyle medicine interventions. *Microorganisms*. 2018;6(2):35.

401. McKeown NM, Fahey GC, Slavin J, van der Kamp JW. Fibre intake for optimal health: how can healthcare professionals support people to reach dietary recommendations? *BMJ*. 2022;378:e054370.

402. McRorie J. Clinical data support that psyllium is not fermented in the gut. *Am J Gastroenterol*. 2013;108(9):1541.

403. Fibersol. Reliability you can count on. Accessed September 15, 2024. https://www.fibersol.com/about-fibersol/trusted-history

404. Fibersol. Innovation=Fibersol® advantage. Accessed September 15, 2024. https://www.fibersol.com/innovation

405. Qin W, Ying W, Hamaker B, Zhang G. Slow digestion-oriented dietary strategy to sustain the secretion of GLP-1 for improved glucose homeostasis. *Compr Rev Food Sci Food Saf*. 2021;20(5):5173–96.

406. McCarty MF, DiNicolantonio JJ. Acarbose, lente carbohydrate, and prebiotics promote metabolic health and longevity by stimulating intestinal production of GLP-1. *Open Heart*. 2015;2(1):e000205.

407. Dalsgaard NB, Gasbjerg LS, Hansen LS, et al. The role of GLP-1 in the postprandial effects of acarbose in type 2 diabetes. *Eur J Endocrinol*. 2021;184(3):383–94.

408. Remde A, DeTurk SN, Almardini A, Steiner L, Wojda T. Plant-predominant eating patterns—how effective are they for treating obesity and related cardiometabolic health outcomes?—a systematic review. *Nutr Rev*. 2022;80(5):1094–104.

409. McCarty MF, DiNicolantonio JJ. Acarbose, lente carbohydrate, and prebiotics promote metabolic health and longevity by stimulating intestinal production of GLP-1. *Open Heart*. 2015;2(1):e000205.

410. Bajka BH, Pinto AM, Perez-Moral N, et al. Enhanced secretion of satiety-promoting gut hormones in healthy humans after consumption of white bread enriched with cellular chickpea flour: a randomized crossover study. *Am J Clin Nutr*. 2023;117(3):477–89.

411. Mollard RC, Luhovyy BL, Panahi S, Nunez M, Hanley A, Anderson GH. Regular consumption of pulses for 8 weeks reduces metabolic syndrome risk factors in overweight and obese adults. *Br J Nutr*. 2012;108 Suppl 1:S111–22.

412. Oliveira D, Nilsson A. Effects of dark-chocolate on appetite variables and glucose tolerance: a 4 week randomised crossover intervention in healthy middle aged subjects. *J Funct Foods*. 2017;37:390–9.

413. Juntunen KS, Niskanen LK, Liukkonen KH, Poutanen KS, Holst JJ, Mykkänen HM. Postprandial glucose, insulin, and incretin responses to grain products in healthy subjects. *Am J Clin Nutr*. 2002;75(2):254–62.

414. Mofidi A, Ferraro ZM, Stewart KA, et al. The acute impact of ingestion of sourdough and whole-grain breads on blood glucose, insulin, and incretins in overweight and obese men. *J Nutr Metab*. 2012;2012:184710.

415. Hassanzadeh-Rostami Z, Ghobadi S, Faghih S. Effects of whole grain intake on glucagon-like peptide 1 and glucose-dependent insulinotropic peptide: a systematic review and meta-analysis. *Nutr Rev.* 2023;81(4):384–96.

416. Willett WC. The dietary pyramid: does the foundation need repair? *Am J Clin Nutr.* 1998;68(2):218–9.

417. Nilsson AC, Ostman EM, Holst JJ, Björck IME. Including indigestible carbohydrates in the evening meal of healthy subjects improves glucose tolerance, lowers inflammatory markers, and increases satiety after a subsequent standardized breakfast. *J Nutr.* 2008;138(4):732–9.

418. Johansson EV, Nilsson AC, Östman EM, Björck IME. Effects of indigestible carbohydrates in barley on glucose metabolism, appetite and voluntary food intake over 16 h in healthy adults. *Nutr J.* 2013;12:46.

419. Nilsson AC, Johansson-Boll EV, Björck IME. Increased gut hormones and insulin sensitivity index following a 3-d intervention with a barley kernel-based product: a randomised cross-over study in healthy middle-aged subjects. *Br J Nutr.* 2015;114(6):899–907.

420. Sandberg JC, Björck IME, Nilsson AC. Rye-based evening meals favorably affected glucose regulation and appetite variables at the following breakfast: a randomized controlled study in healthy subjects. *PLoS One.* 2016;11(3):e0151985.

421. Rebello CJ, Greenway FL. Reward-induced eating: therapeutic approaches to addressing food cravings. *Adv Ther.* 2016;33(11):1853–66.

422. Erlanson-Albertsson C, Albertsson PÅ. The use of green leaf membranes to promote appetite control, suppress hedonic hunger and loose [sic] body weight. *Plant Foods Hum Nutr.* 2015;70(3):281–90.

423. Stenblom EL. *Intestinal regulation of hunger and reward. Studies with thylakoids.* Dissertation. Lund University: Faculty of Medicine; 2016.

424. Erlanson-Albertsson C, Albertsson PÅ. The use of green leaf membranes to promote appetite control, suppress hedonic hunger and loose [sic] body weight. *Plant Foods Hum Nutr.* 2015;70(3):281–90.

425. Stenblom EL, Montelius C, Östbring K, et al. Supplementation by thylakoids to a high carbohydrate meal decreases feelings of hunger, elevates CCK levels and prevents postprandial hypoglycaemia in overweight women. *Appetite.* 2013;68:118–23.

426. Rebello CJ, Chu J, Beyl R, Edwall D, Erlanson-Albertsson C, Greenway FL. Acute effects of a spinach extract rich in thylakoids on satiety: a randomized controlled crossover trial. *J Am Coll Nutr.* 2015;34(6):470–7.

427. Stenblom EL, Egecioglu E, Landin-Olsson M, Erlanson-Albertsson C. Consumption of thylakoid-rich spinach extract reduces hunger, increases satiety and reduces cravings for palatable food in overweight women. *Appetite.* 2015;91:209–19.

428. Gustafsson K, Asp NG, Hagander B, Nyman M. Satiety effects of spinach in mixed meals: comparison with other vegetables. Satiety effects of spinach in mixed meals: comparison with other vegetables. *Int J Food Sci Nutr.* 1995;46(4):327–34.

429. Amirinejad A, Heshmati J, Shidfar F. Effects of thylakoid intake on appetite and weight loss: a systematic review. *J Diabetes Metab Disord.* 2020;19(1):565–73.

430. Stenblom EL, Egecioglu E, Landin-Olsson M, Erlanson-Albertsson C. Consumption of thylakoid-rich spinach extract reduces hunger, increases satiety and reduces cravings for palatable food in overweight women. *Appetite.* 2015;91:209–19.

431. Erlanson-Albertsson C, Albertsson PÅ. The use of green leaf membranes to promote appetite control, suppress hedonic hunger and loose [sic] body weight. *Plant Foods Hum Nutr*. 2015;70(3):281–90.

432. Stenblom EL, Egecioglu E, Landin-Olsson M, Erlanson-Albertsson C. Consumption of thylakoid-rich spinach extract reduces hunger, increases satiety and reduces cravings for palatable food in overweight women. *Appetite*. 2015;91:209–19.

433. Montelius C, Erlandsson D, Vitija E, Stenblom EL, Egecioglu E, Erlanson-Albertsson C. Body weight loss, reduced urge for palatable food and increased release of GLP-1 through daily supplementation with green-plant membranes for three months in overweight women. *Appetite*. 2014;81:295–304.

434. Montelius C, Erlandsson D, Vitija E, Stenblom EL, Egecioglu E, Erlanson-Albertsson C. Body weight loss, reduced urge for palatable food and increased release of GLP-1 through daily supplementation with green-plant membranes for three months in overweight women. *Appetite*. 2014;81:295–304.

435. Stenblom ES, Montelius C, Erlandsson D, et al. Decreased urge for palatable food after a two month dietary intervention with green-plant membranes in overweight women. *J Obes Weight Loss Ther*. 2014;4:4.

436. EFSA Panel on Nutrition, Novel Foods and Food Allergens (NDA), Turck D, Bohn T, et al. Appethyl® and reduction of body weight: evaluation of a health claim pursuant to Article 13(5) of Regulation (Ec) No 1924/2006. *EFSA J*. 2023;21(10):e08239.

437. Pourteymour Fard Tabrizi F, Abbasalizad Farhangi M, Vaezi M, Hemmati S. Changes of body composition and circulating neopterin, omentin-1, and chemerin in response to thylakoid-rich spinach extract with a hypocaloric diet in obese women with polycystic ovary syndrome: a randomized controlled trial. *Phytother Res*. 2021;35(5):2594–606.

438. Stenblom EL, Montelius C, Östbring K, et al. Supplementation by thylakoids to a high carbohydrate meal decreases feelings of hunger, elevates CCK levels and prevents postprandial hypoglycaemia in overweight women. *Appetite*. 2013;68:118–23.

439. Erlanson-Albertsson C, Albertsson PÅ. The use of green leaf membranes to promote appetite control, suppress hedonic hunger and loose [sic] body weight. *Plant Foods Hum Nutr*. 2015;70(3):281–90.

440. Pourteymour Fard Tabrizi F, Abbasalizad Farhangi M. A systematic review of the potential effects of thylakoids in the management of obesity and its related issues. *Food Rev Int*. 2021;37(5):469–90.

441. Pourteymour Fard Tabrizi F, Abbasalizad Farhangi M. A systematic review of the potential effects of thylakoids in the management of obesity and its related issues. *Food Rev Int*. 2021;37(5):469–90.

442. Rebello CJ, O'Neil CE, Greenway FL. Gut fat signaling and appetite control with special emphasis on the effect of thylakoids from spinach on eating behavior. *Int J Obes (Lond)*. 2015;39(12):1679–88.

443. Erlanson-Albertsson C, Albertsson PÅ. The use of green leaf membranes to promote appetite control, suppress hedonic hunger and loose [sic] body weight. *Plant Foods Hum Nutr*. 2015;70(3):281–90.

444. Östbring K, Rayner M, Sjöholm I, et al. The effect of heat treatment of thylakoids on their ability to inhibit *in vitro* lipase/co-lipase activity. *Food Funct*. 2014;5(9):2157–65.

445. Estebaranz F, Galbany J, Martínez L, Turbón D, Pérez-Pérez A. Buccal dental microwear analyses support greater specialization in consumption of hard foodstuffs for *Australopithecus anamensis*. *J Anthropol Sci*. 2012;90:163–85.

446. Roberts JL, Moreau R. Functional properties of spinach (*Spinacia oleracea* L.) phytochemicals and bioactives. *Food Funct*. 2016;7(8):3337–53.

447. Gertsch J. The metabolic plant feedback hypothesis: how plant secondary metabolites nonspecifically impact human health. *Planta Med*. 2016;82(11–12):920–9.

448. Östbring K, Sjöholm I, Sörenson H, Ekholm A, Erlanson-Albertsson C, Rayner M. Characteristics and functionality of appetite-reducing thylakoid powders produced by three different drying processes. *J Sci Food Agric*. 2018;98(4):1554–65.

449. Lewis KH, Moore JB, Ard JD. Game changers: do new medications make lifestyle-based treatment of obesity obsolete? *Obesity (Silver Spring)*. 2024;32(2):237–9.

450. Mozaffarian D. GLP-1 agonists for obesity—a new recipe for success? *JAMA*. 2024;331(12):1007–8.

451. 60 Minutes Overtime. S55 E16: Doctors explain how Wegovy and Ozempic work. Paramount. Aired January 1, 2023. Accessed September 15, 2025. https://www.paramountplus.com/shows/video/jS8m7bZVPSiYWOcXcHn4107Km6_NTtie/?ftag=CNM-00-10abb6c

452. Lexchin J, Mintzes B. Semaglutide: a new drug for the treatment of obesity. *Drug Ther Bull*. 2023;61(12):182–8.

453. Lexchin J, Mintzes B. Semaglutide: a new drug for the treatment of obesity. *Drug Ther Bull*. 2023;61(12):182–8.

454. Wilding JPH, Mooney V, Pile R. Should obesity be recognised as a disease? *BMJ*. Published online July 17, 2019:l4258.

455. Swinburn BA, Sacks G, Hall KD, et al. The global obesity pandemic: shaped by global drivers and local environments. *Lancet*. 2011;378(9793):804–14.

456. Rodgers A, Woodward A, Swinburn B, Dietz WH. Prevalence trends tell us what did not precipitate the US obesity epidemic. *Lancet Public Health*. 2018;3(4):e162–3.

457. Cohen DA. Neurophysiological pathways to obesity: below awareness and beyond individual control. *Diabetes*. 2008;57(7):1768–73.

458. Rodgers A, Woodward A, Swinburn B, Dietz WH. Prevalence trends tell us what did not precipitate the US obesity epidemic. *Lancet Public Health*. 2018;3(4):e162–3.

459. Swinburn BA, Sacks G, Hall KD, et al. The global obesity pandemic: shaped by global drivers and local environments. *Lancet*. 2011;378(9793):804–14.

460. Waynforth D. Evolution, obesity, and why children so often choose the unhealthy eating option. *Med Hypotheses*. 2010;74(5):934–6.

461. Rutter H. Where next for obesity? *Lancet*. 2011;378(9793):746–7.

462. Rutter H. Where next for obesity? *Lancet*. 2011;378(9793):746–7.

463. Fryar CD, Carroll MD, Afful J. Prevalence of overweight, obesity, and severe obesity among adults aged 20 and over: United States, 1960–1962 through 2017–2018. National Center for Health Statistics. CDC.gov. January 29, 2021. Accessed September 15, 2024. https://www.cdc.gov/nchs/data/hestat/obesity-adult-17-18/obesity-adult.htm

464. Egger G, Swinburn B. An "ecological" approach to the obesity pandemic. *BMJ*. 1997;315(7106):477–80.

465. Dowsett GKC, Yeo GSH. Are GLP-1R agonists the long-sought-after panacea for obesity? *Trends Mol Med*. 2023;29(10):777–9.

466. Klitzman R, Greenberg H. Anti-obesity medications: ethical, policy, and public health concerns. *Hastings Cent Rep*. 2024;54(3):6–10.

467. McCartney M. Semaglutide: should the media slim down its enthusiasm? *BMJ*. 2023;380:624.

468. Battle EK, Brownell KD. Confronting a rising tide of eating disorders and obesity: treatment vs. prevention and policy. *Addict Behav*. 1996;21(6):755–65.

469. Osmick MJ, Wilson M. Social determinants of health—relevant history, a call to action, an organization's transformational story, and what can employers do? *Am J Health Promot*. 2020;34(2):219–24.

470. About CDC. Social determinants of health (SDOH). CDC.gov. January 17, 2024. Accessed September 15, 2024. https://www.cdc.gov/about/priorities/why-is-addressing-sdoh-important.html

471. Chetty R, Stepner M, Abraham S, et al. The association between income and life expectancy in the United States, 2001-2014. *JAMA*. 2016;315(16):1750–66.

472. West R, Marteau T. Commentary on Casswell (2013): the commercial determinants of health. *Addiction*. 2013;108(4):686–87.

473. Millar JS. The corporate determinants of health: how big business affects our health, and the need for government action! *Can J Public Health*. 2013;104(4):e327–9.

474. West R, Marteau T. Commentary on Casswell (2013): the commercial determinants of health. *Addiction*. 2013;108(4):686–7.

475. Drug and Therapeutics Bulletin. About. BMJ Journals. Accessed September 16, 2024. https://dtb.bmj.com/pages/about

476. Lexchin J, Mintzes B. Semaglutide: a new drug for the treatment of obesity. *Drug Ther Bull*. 2023;61(12):182–8.

477. McCartney M. Semaglutide: should the media slim down its enthusiasm? *BMJ*. 2023;380:624.

478. Onakpoya IJ, Heneghan CJ, Aronson JK. Post-marketing withdrawal of anti-obesity medicinal products because of adverse drug reactions: a systematic review. *BMC Med*. 2016;14(1):191.

479. Mullard A. Mediator scandal rocks French medical community. *Lancet*. 2011;377(9769):890–2.

480. Chawla A, Carls G, Deng E, Tuttle E. The expected net present value of developing weight management drugs in the context of drug safety litigation. *PharmacoEconomics*. 2015;33(7):749–63.

481. Reuters. French drugmaker Servier ordered to pay $471 million for Mediator scandal. Reuters.com. December 20, 2023. Accessed September 16, 2024. https://www.reuters.com/business/healthcare-pharmaceuticals/french-drugmaker-servier-ordered-pay-471-million-mediator-scandal-2023-12-20/

482. Mullard A. Mediator scandal rocks French medical community. *Lancet*. 2011;377(9769):890-2.

483. Mullard A. Mediator scandal rocks French medical community. *Lancet*. 2011;377(9769):890-2.

484. Reuters. French drugmaker Servier ordered to pay $471 million for Mediator scandal. Reuters.com. December 20, 2023. Accessed September 16, 2024. https://www.reuters.com/business/healthcare-pharmaceuticals/french-drugmaker-servier-ordered-pay-471-million-mediator-scandal-2023-12-20/

485. Mozaffarian D. GLP-1 agonists for obesity—a new recipe for success? *JAMA*. 2024;331(12):1007-8.

486. Prospective Studies Collaboration, Whitlock G, Lewington S, et al. Body-mass index and cause-specific mortality in 900 000 adults: collaborative analyses of 57 prospective studies. *Lancet*. 2009;373(9669):1083–96.

487. Dapre E. Are GLP-1 agonists the answer to our obesity epidemic? *Br J Gen Pract*. 2023;73(733):365.

488. Di Ciaula A, Portincasa P. Contrasting obesity: is something missing here? *Intern Emerg Med*. 2024;19(2):265–9.

489. Lexchin J, Mintzes B. Semaglutide: a new drug for the treatment of obesity. *Drug Ther Bull*. 2023;61(12):182–8.

490. Prospective Studies Collaboration, Whitlock G, Lewington S, et al. Body-mass index and cause-specific mortality in 900 000 adults: collaborative analyses of 57 prospective studies. *Lancet*. 2009;373(9669):1083–16.

491. Gibbons C, Blundell J, Tetens Hoff S, Dahl K, Bauer R, Baekdal T. Effects of oral semaglutide on energy intake, food preference, appetite, control of eating and body weight in subjects with type 2 diabetes. *Diabetes Obes Metab*. 2021;23(2):581–8.

492. Blundell J, Finlayson G, Axelsen M, et al. Effects of once-weekly semaglutide on appetite, energy intake, control of eating, food preference and body weight in subjects with obesity. *Diabetes Obes Metab*. 2017;19(9):1242–51.

493. Lewis KH, Moore JB, Ard JD. Game changers: do new medications make lifestyle-based treatment of obesity obsolete? *Obesity (Silver Spring)*. 2024;32(2):237–9.

494. Hall KD. Physiology of the weight-loss plateau in response to diet restriction, GLP-1 receptor agonism, and bariatric surgery. *Obesity (Silver Spring)*. 2024;32(6):1163–8.

495. Duncan KH, Bacon JA, Weinsier RL. The effects of high and low energy density diets on satiety, energy intake, and eating time of obese and nonobese subjects. *Am J Clin Nutr*. 1983;37(5):763–7.

496. Chen Y, Henson S, Jackson AB, Richards JS. Obesity intervention in persons with spinal cord injury. *Spinal Cord*. 2006;44(2):82–91.

497. Wright N, Wilson L, Smith M, Duncan B, McHugh P. The BROAD study: a randomised controlled trial using a whole food plant-based diet in the community for obesity, ischaemic heart disease or diabetes. *Nutr Diabetes*. 2017;7(3):e256.

498. Barnard ND, Kahleova H. For appetite control, drugs vs diet. *Am J Med*. 2024;137(3):198–9.

499. Kahleova H, Sutton M, Maracine C, et al. Vegan diet and food costs among adults with overweight: a secondary analysis of a randomized clinical trial. *JAMA Netw Open*. 2023;6(9):e2332106.

500. Kamakura R, Raza GS, Sodum N, Lehto VP, Kovalainen M, Herzig KH. Colonic delivery of nutrients for sustained and prolonged release of gut peptides: a novel strategy for appetite management. *Mol Nutr Food Res*. 2022;66(19):e2200192.

501. McKeown NM, Fahey GC, Slavin J, van der Kamp JW. Fibre intake for optimal health: how can healthcare professionals support people to reach dietary recommendations? *BMJ*. 2022;378:e054370.

502. Wright N, Wilson L, Smith M, Duncan B, McHugh P. The BROAD study: a randomised controlled trial using a whole food plant-based diet in the community for obesity, ischaemic heart disease or diabetes. *Nutr Diabetes*. 2017;7(3):e256.

INDEX

Made in United States
Troutdale, OR
10/30/2024